# Breast Cancer Mimics

**Urszula Wegner, MD**
Consultant Breast Radiologist
Kettering General Hospital
Kettering, United Kingdom

**Chitrangada Singh, MD**
Honorary Fellow
Department of Breast Imaging
Norfolk and Norwich University Hospital
Norfolk, United Kingdom

Thieme
Delhi • Stuttgart • New York • Rio de Janeiro

Publishing Director: Ritu Sharma
Development Editor: Dr Ambika Kapoor
Director-Editorial Services: Rachna Sinha
Project Manager: Gaurav Prabhu
Vice President, Sales and Marketing:
Arun Kumar Majji
Managing Director & CEO: Ajit Kohli

Thieme Medical and Scientific Publishers Private
Limited.
A - 12, Second Floor, Sector - 2, Noida - 201 301,
Uttar Pradesh, India, +911204556600
Email: customerservice@thieme.in
www.thieme.in

Cover design: Thieme Publishing Group
Typesetting by RECTO Graphics, India

Printed in India by Nutech Print Services

5 4 3 2 1

ISBN: 978-93-88257-94-7

In fond memory of:

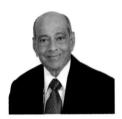

Prof. Dr. Mukund Sadashiv Joshi (1942–2020)

The father of Indian Ultrasound.
Hon. Member of Radiological Society of North America and
American College of Radiology.

A visionary and true teacher who raised the levels of numerous radiologists by
inculcating in them the finest of radiological knowledge.

# Contents

# Foreword

It gives me immense pleasure to introduce this book intended for breast imaging specialists, breast surgeons, radiologists, radiology residents, fellows, and physicians practicing breast imaging. Both experts and beginners can use this excellent book for differential diagnosis of breast cancer mimics. This fills a gap in series of breast imaging as this book is the first of its kind.

Dr Wegner and Dr Singh have compiled an excellent collection of entities that closely mimic breast cancer but are benign. This will help the reader to develop a well-thought-of differential for breast cancer and help to appropriate triaging of the patients.

The book is well organized and easy to read with numerous examples and concepts. The chapters are uniformly structured, each section is richly illustrated, including multimodality imaging and histopathology correlation where appropriate. Each chapter has a quiz in the format of multiple-choice questions and answers for the reader to test the knowledge gained. This feature of self-assessment is a welcome change which is not seen in many other books on the same subject.

*Breast Cancer Mimics* meets the needs of its intended audience and is the book I would recommend for all breast imagers, radiology residents, fellows, and physicians practicing breast imaging, and for departmental libraries.

**Vikram Dogra, MD, FAIUM, FSRU, FSAR,**
Professor of Radiology and Biomedical Engineering
Director Division of Ultrasound
Department of Imaging Science
University of Rochester
New York, New York, USA

# Foreword

Mark Twain once said, "Education is the path from cocky ignorance to miserable uncertainty."

Who could possibly understand this better than a breast imager, for whom truth is sometimes stranger than fiction!

Nonetheless, it is the duty of the educator to fill in the void. And that is precisely the void that this excellent compilation on breast cancer mimics fills in! It gives me immense pleasure to introduce *Breast Cancer Mimics*, a topic which has not been addressed in any other book.

The highlights of this book are the well-illustrated images along with diagrammatic comparisons of benign conditions with similar-appearing malignancies. The book boasts of a strong compilation of over 100 cases with multimodality imaging and histopathology correlation.

There are comprehensive teaching points at the end of each chapter and multiple choice questions to assess knowledge gained.

Dr Wegner and Dr Singh have indeed struck a century in their maiden innings. These dynamic radiologists have contributed in an area of breast imaging where others have not ventured.

I strongly recommend this book to radiologists-in-training, fellows, general radiologists, breast imaging specialists, breast surgeons, and every single reader who wishes to excel in the art and science of breast imaging.

**Shilpa Lad, MD**
Consultant Breast Imaging & Interventions
NM Medical Center, Mumbai, India;
Sub Specialty Head (SSH)
Breast Imaging & Interventions
Indian College of Radiological Imaging (ICRI);
Former Staff Radiologist & Assistant Professor
Section of Breast Imaging
The Ottawa Hospital, University of Ottawa,
Ottawa, Canada

# Preface

> "[Being a doctor] offers the most complete and constant union of
> those three qualities which have the greatest charm for pure and
> active minds – novelty, utility, and charity."
>
> —Sir James Paget (1814–1899)

We are glad to introduce the first edition of this book, which is completely based on conditions that look similar to breast cancer on routine imaging modalities such as ultrasound and mammography, which are an essential element of most breast cancer screening programs.

As you flip through the pages of this book, you will discover categorically placed benign findings in breast patients, which often have the effect of puzzling us as we move along the cancer pathway. The categorization will help the reader to not just appreciate the findings but also develop an orientation regarding the group of patients which best fits the category, thereby progressing with a broader perception of diagnosis.

Each topic has been supplemented by radiological findings, and correlating them with histology will provide confidence for discussion and defend their perception in multidisciplinary teams. Various high-resolution images of even the rarest of rare findings have been discussed in the book to plan for the unexpected cases with the help of radiologists and pathologists around the globe.

Practically relevant summarized text and comparison images also help the radiologist focus on the points of interest when comparing such close differentials. Each chapter is followed by a short summary quiz for self-assessment purpose. Adequate explanations have also been included to cater to inquisitive minds.

Urszula Wegner is thankful to her husband Jay, and their little daughter Laura, for supporting her through all these months of travelling, compiling cases and materializing them, and sacrificing their family time.

Chitrangada Singh is thankful to her husband, Dr Lokesh Sharoff, and her family for providing the book with feedback and suggestions and motivating her to pursue this project with unwavering dedication from the time of its conception.

We express our sincere thanks to the editorial team of Thieme Books for aiding us through the process of book publishing, sorting and discussing the numerous details, and conducting editing sessions which helped us in shaping this book.

**Urszula Wegner, MD**
**Chitrangada Singh, MD**

# Acknowledgments

We would like to express our deepest appreciation to all the professionals who supported us and provided us with the golden opportunity of finalizing this wonderful project. This international collaboration between medical experts belonging to various countries in the field of radiology and breast imaging is also an example of radiology beyond borders, which enabled us to cover such rare and regional diseases with ease.

It was an honor to share this unique international collection of cases with dedicated radiologists, pathologists, and radiographers who have offered us generous support by way of sharing with us advances in the field.

Also, we would like to thank all our mentors and teachers who empowered us and kept us motivated to accomplish what they trained us for.

We are particularly grateful to the following reputed professionals for their extraordinary support and motivation:

**Sabine Balschat, MD, PhD**
Consultant Radiologist
Dietrich-Bonhoeffer-Klinikum
Neubrandenburg, Germany

**Carmel Ann Daly, FFR (RCSI)**
Consultant Radiologist
University Hospital Waterford
Waterford City, Republic of Ireland

**Michal Kujach, MD**
Consultant Pathologist
Public Hospital Koscierzyna
Koscierzyna, Poland

**Lavina Laungani, MD**
Junior Consultant Histopathologist
Prince Aly Khan Hospital
Mumbai, India

**Rajesh Logasundaram, FRCPath**
Consultant Pathologist
Norfolk and Norwich University Hospitals
Norfolk, United Kingdom

**Joseph Murphy, FRCPath**
Consultant Pathologist
Norfolk and Norwich University Hospitals
Norfolk, United Kingdom

**Nirali Patel, MD**
Resident Radiologist
D. Y. Patil Hospital
Mumbai, India

**Prof Anthony Ryan, FFRCSI, FRCR**
Consultant Radiologist
University Hospital Waterford
Waterford City, Republic of Ireland

**Nigam Shah, MD**
Consultant Pathologist
University Hospital Waterford
Waterford City, Republic of Ireland

**Suneet Singh, MD**
Fellow in Cytopathology
King Edward Memorial Hospital
Mumbai, India

**Swati Singh, MD**
Consultant Pathologist
Apex Hospital and Cancer Care
Varanasi, India


We wish to extend special thanks to the following reputed individuals, who are enthusiastic and dedicated consultant breast radiographers in their own right:

**Sarah Rainford, MSc, BSc (Hons)**
Consultant Breast Radiographer
Kettering General Hospital
Kettering, United Kingdom

**Karen Wren, MSc, DCR (r)**
Consultant Breast Radiographer
Kettering General Hospital
Kettering, United Kingdom


We greatly thank all of you for your outstanding work which made this dream a reality!

**Urszula Wegner, MD**
**Chitrangada Singh, MD**

# About the Authors

**Urszula Wegner** is an experienced consultant radiologist who is recognized for her aptitude in research conducted on breast imaging. She has worked across the UK and Europe in public and NHS hospitals, yielding a strong academic and professional development record. This has included a Breast Imaging Observership in Germany and fellowships in UK and Ireland, National Diploma in Radiology & Diagnostic Imaging, and EDIR certificate. Urszula's clinical work includes screening and diagnostic mammography, diagnostic breast ultrasound, screening and diagnostic breast MRI, all the while ensuring complete accuracy and attention to detail. Her research interests include mammographic screening and breast cancer risk assessment; early breast cancer detection and extent of disease evaluation using contrast-enhanced mammography and MRI. She has been an invited presenter at Radiological Society of North America (RSNA) 2019 and also authored European Society of Radiology learning modules and publications in reputable international journals. Urszula's key expertise is founded Europe-wide, developing key networks within the medical field; maintaining high standards, passion, and fulfilling her career in breast radiology.

**Chitrangada Singh,** after graduating at the top of her class from D. Y. Patil Hospital and Research Centre with a Gold medal distinction in MD Radio-diagnosis, had the opportunity to work under the mentorship of some of the leading radiologists in the city and country.

Her academic inclination and various award-winning presentations at conferences in Radiology paved the way toward bagging the award scholarship in Advanced Breast Imaging by European Society of Radiology at the Norwich and Norfolk University Hospitals, UK. During this time, she was exposed to a wide array of breast interventions, innovative methods of localizations of non-palpable breast masses, contrast-enhanced mammography, MRI, and professional staging with multidisciplinary correlations, forging a strong reputation and high standards of professional excellence. In 2019, her efforts were again appreciated by the RSNA in the form of a travel grant and conference invitation.

Chitrangada has numerous publications in national and international journals, including spectrum of original articles, guidelines, and case reports. She has been an invited speaker at the oncology conference and ultrasound conference in Australia, UK, and Dubai.

She has also coauthored breast imaging e-learning modules for the European Society of Radiology.

# Introduction

Breast imaging as a subspecialty is still evolving. Multi-country screening programs and guidelines are being updated every year with knowledge being expanded and new techniques emerging. However, there are still diverse nonmalignant entities that create a mind block on available imaging modalities. Many of these uncommon conditions may be easily mistaken for breast cancer; thus, it was imperative to highlight these entities and present the subgroups of abnormalities imitating malignancy.

Misleading mimickers can be categorized in the setting of inflammatory conditions, proliferative disorders, changes secondary to autoimmune and metabolic diseases, lesions of neural origin, or vascular anomalies.

Complications of long-standing diabetes in breast radiology will also be highlighted in detail as it lacks awareness and, hence, easily confuses young breast radiologists.

Diagnostic pearls and challenges that have been observed by breast radiologists over the years have all been compiled in this book. The comparison slides effortlessly help in identifying the subtle features which distinguish the mimickers from the neoplastic lesions.

The language is simple yet interesting. The comprehensive review will imbue confidence in the readers, offering them some of the most unique and rare breast cancer mimics from across the world apart from the routine masqueraders.

We will review a unique and interesting international collection of cases with their imaging spectrum with diagnostic pearls.

These challenging conditions can be categorized into subgroups, namely,

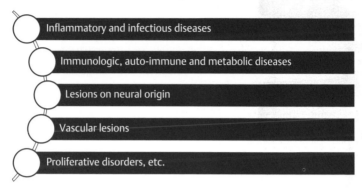

Inflammatory and infectious diseases

Immunologic, auto-immune and metabolic diseases

Lesions on neural origin

Vascular lesions

Proliferative disorders, etc.

We would also take this opportunity to emphasize that imaging cannot always establish a definitive diagnosis in isolation and having an open mind with a multidisciplinary approach and prompt biopsy becomes obligatory to avoid negligence. This book provides pathological correlation and microscopic pictures to reinstate this concept in the mind of the reader.

The self-assessment part is associated with developmental feedback which is designed to enhance your knowledge and help you recapitulate the potential future challenges.

We wish you all the best, as you embark on this journey toward gaining a better understanding of breast radiology.

# Chapter 1

## Inflammatory and Infectious Diseases

# Inflammatory and Infectious Diseases

---

## Learning Objectives:

1. To provide fundamentals of various inflammatory and infectious conditions that can imitate malignant processes with regard to radiological or physical examination.

2. To highlight the characteristic imaging features which enable the diagnosis and help exclude malignancies.

3. To reinforce the knowledge during subsequent comprehensive quiz with developmental feedback.

---

## Introduction

Various inflammatory and infectious conditions may cause diagnostic dilemma and can possess interesting and unusual imaging features which can mislead dedicated breast imaging experts regardless of experience. We will discuss some of the most challenging diseases including examples of tuberculous mastitis, idiopathic granulomatous mastitis, silicone mastitis, infective mastitis, or parasitic infestation of the breast.

## Tuberculous Mastitis

Tuberculous mastitis is one of the differentials regarding the imaging spectrum of granulomatous mastitis and is caused by Mycobacterium tuberculosis. Breast tuberculosis was first reported by Sir Astley Cooper in 1829.

It is one of the rare manifestations of the extrapulmonary tuberculosis.

Breast tuberculosis is common in females of reproductive age. However, the incidence is rare in older females and male breast. Usually one breast is involved. The regular symptoms of weight loss and anorexia may be absent in patients with breast tuberculosis.

One of the most sensitive confirmation tests is polymerase chain reaction (PCR) from the aspirate. The gold standard still remains Ziehl Nielsen staining of aspirate to demonstrate casseating granulomas with Langhan's giant cells (granulomas on **Fig. 1.1a**).

Treatment consists of standard antituberculosis therapy. However, surgical interventions may be considered in cases of poor response to treatment or extensive, symptomatic disease.

It can present as a solitary, atypical breast mass (**Fig. 1.1b–e**) or may be associated with breast edema or axillary lymphadenopathy.

Fistulae or sinus tract formation is not unusual. However, it may be seen secondary to drainage or surgical excision.

Differential diagnoses and diagnostic dilemmas in the setting of granulomatous inflammation can be secondary to several other conditions such as sarcoidosis, granulomatosis with polyangiitis (formerly known as Wegener's granulomatosis), or simply foreign body reaction. Granulomatous mastitis can also be idiopathic.

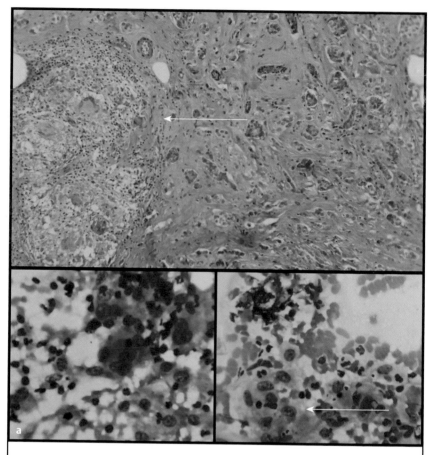

**Fig. 1.1 (a)** Granulomas in the setting of tuberculous mastitis (*arrows*). Histology shows casseating granulomas with characteristic central necrosis surrounded by Langhan's giant cells and epithelioid cells. The infiltrates show lymphocytic predominance.

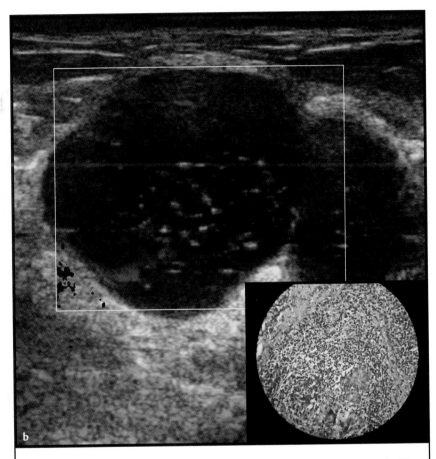

**Fig. 1.1 (b)** Mammary tuberculosis. A 35-year-old female with a history of a palpable and tender breast lump. Ultrasound revealed a complex mass with both solid-appearing and more fluid-like components. Histology confirmed tuberculous mastitis (*inset*).

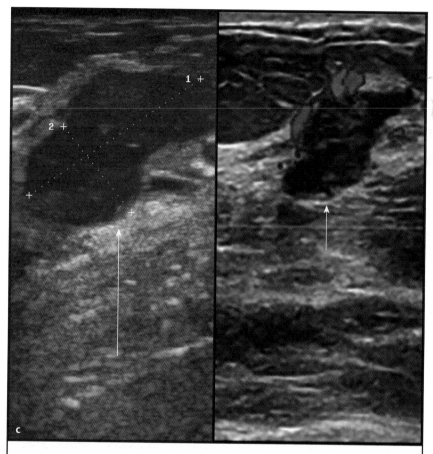

**Fig. 1.1 (c)** Diagnostic challenges on sonography. Comparison slide shows mammary tuberculosis (*long arrow*) and intracystic papillary carcinoma (*short arrow*). Please note that tuberculosis and malignancy may have shared imaging features and present as complex masses, with both solid-appearing and fluid-like components (please see explanations on **Fig. 1.1d**).

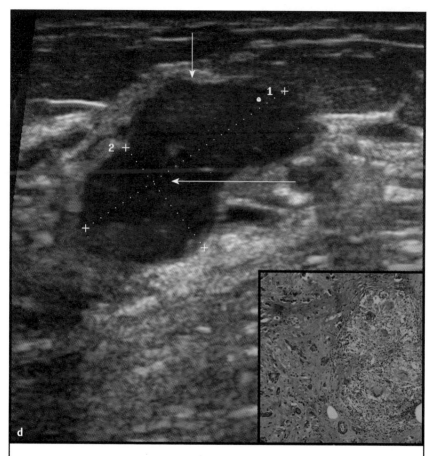

**Fig. 1.1 (d)** Complex mass in the setting of tuberculous mastitis. The presented mass is heterogenous and contains solid-appearing components (*short arrow*) and fluid-like components in the central part (*long arrow*). Associated microphotograph (*inset*).

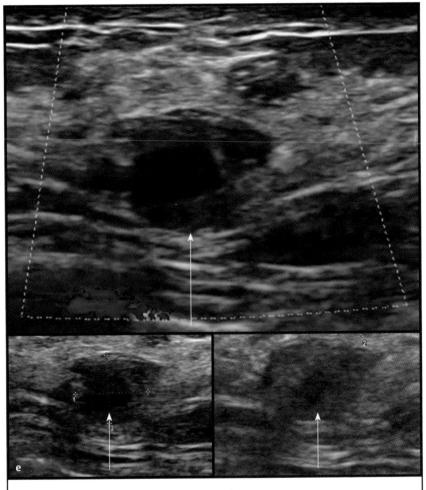

**Fig. 1.1 (e)** Complex masses in the setting of mammary tuberculosis. A 34-year old female patient with a history of tuberculosis and painless long-standing nipple discharge. The presented lesions are heterogenous (*arrows*). These contain both solid-appearing components and fluid-like components in the central parts. Histopathology revealed tuberculous mastitis.

# Idiopathic Granulomatous Mastitis (IGM)

Idiopathic granulomatous mastitis (IGM) is a chronic inflammatory, granulomatous breast disease and often a malignancy mimic. IGM is usually a sterile inflammation which will not respond to empiric antibiotics and can be recurrent.

This condition can not only have bizarre appearances on imaging and radiological findings but also often have shared features with those of breast carcinoma. This type of lobular mastitis was first described by Kesler and Wolloch in 1972.

The initial phase of the disease consists of an acute inflammation which results in an aseptic abscess formation with associated skin thickening and edema of the surrounding tissues.

This is a chronic, recurrent, and self-limiting process which subsequently progresses to fibrosis and the final stage of IGM, with no signs of inflammation on all imaging modalities.

Most common clinical presentation of IGM is as a tender and palpable lump in the unilateral breast (**Fig. 1.2a–c, Fig. 1.3**, and **Fig. 1.4**).

Associated axillary lymphadenopathy often concerns the possibility of malignant pathology with nodal metastases. The lymph nodes are usually nontender on clinical examination.

Sonography usually shows an irregular hypoechoic mass with tubular extension representing the inflammatory process (**Fig. 1.2c** and **Fig. 1.3**). Imaging may be confusing and often labeled as BI-RADS category 4 (compare slides on **Fig. 1.2d** and **Fig. 1.4d**).

Histology may reveal granulomas without central casseation or necrosis. Lymphocytes, plasma cells, and multinucleated giant cells surrounding the lobules (**Fig. 1.3**, *inset*).

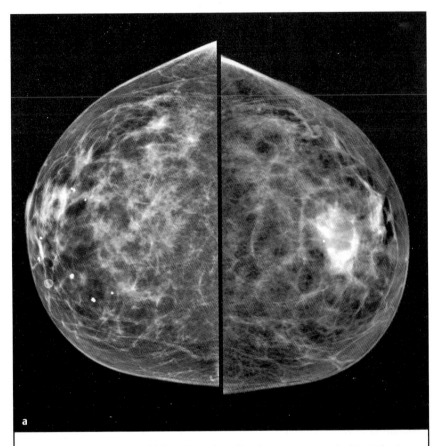

**Fig. 1.2 (a)** A 47-year-old female with a firm breast mass and skin tethering. Mammography revealed an irregular low-density mass within the central left breast.

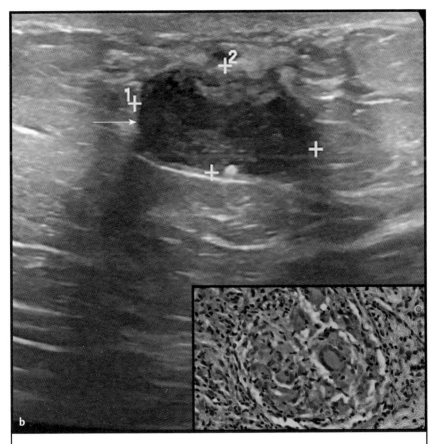

**Fig. 1.2 (b)** The same patient as on **Fig. 1.2a**. Ultrasound scan revealed an irregular heterogenous mass (*arrow*). This contains both solid-appearing components and fluid-like components more centrally. Please see **Fig. 1.2c** with explanations. Associated microphotograph shows a granuloma (*inset*).

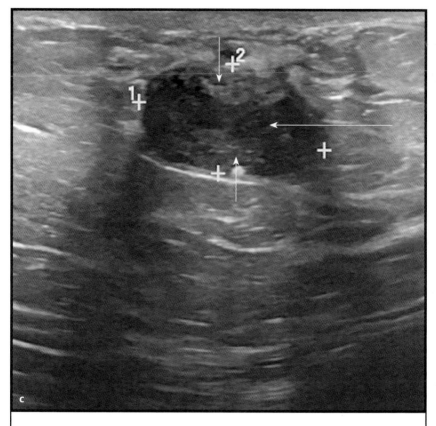

**Fig. 1.2 (c)** The same patient as on **Fig. 1.2a, b**. Complex heterogenous lesion contains both solid-appearing components (*short arrows*) and fluid-like components centrally (*long arrow*).

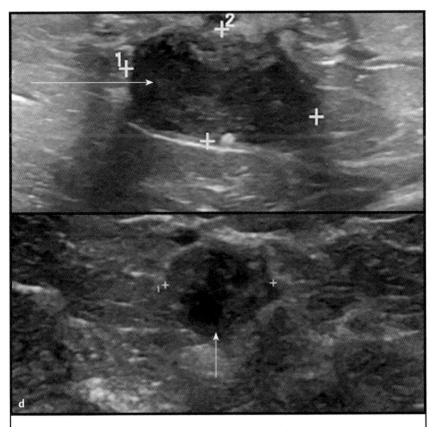

**Fig. 1.2 (d)** Comparison slide shows diagnostic challenges on sonography. Complex masses in the setting of idiopathic granulomatous mastitis (top image, *long arrow*) and invasive mucinous adenocarcinoma (bottom image, *short arrow*). Please note that both malignancy and its mimics have shared imaging features and contain solid-appearing and fluid-like components.

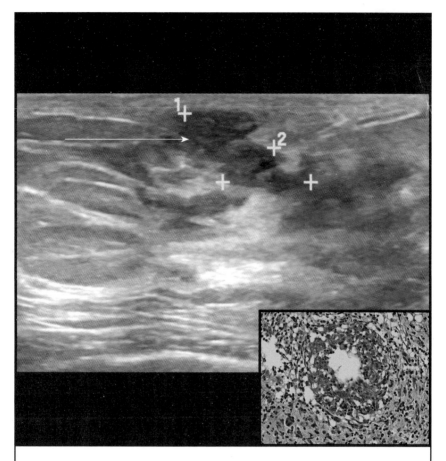

**Fig. 1.3** A 34-year-old patient who presented with a palpable lump at 6 o'clock in the left breast. Ultrasound revealed an irregular hypoechoic mass (*arrow*). Corresponding microphotograph showed a non-casseating granuloma (*inset*).

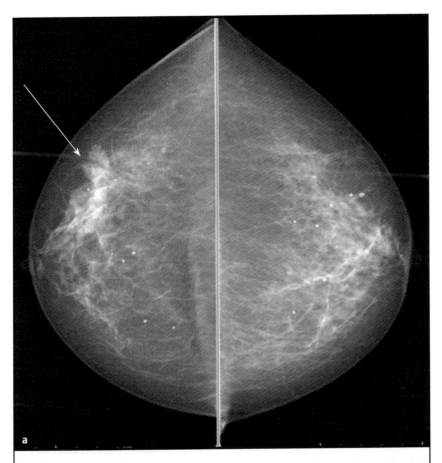

**Fig. 1.4 (a)** A 69-year-old female presented with a firm 2 cm lump with associated skin tethering and erythema. Bilateral mammography, craniocaudal (CC) views shows irregular low-density mass in the setting of granulomatous mastitis (*arrow*). This mass is indistinguishable from carcinoma.

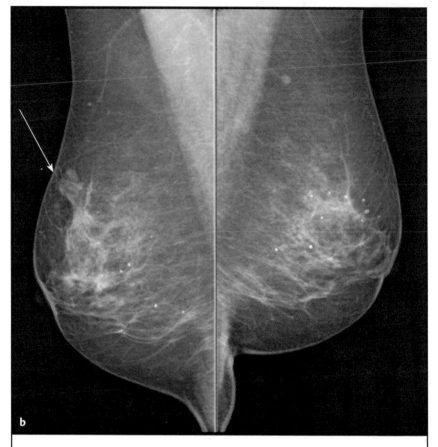

**Fig. 1.4 (b)** The same patient as in Fig. 1.4a. Bilateral mammography, mediolateral–oblique (MLO) views shows granulomatous mastitis within the upper outer right breast (*arrow*).

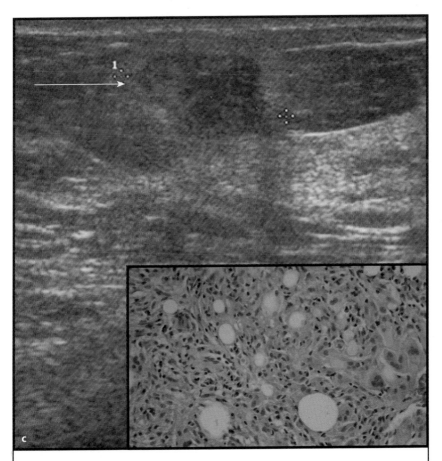

**Fig. 1.4 (c)** The same patient as on **Fig. 1.4a, b**. Subsequent ultrasound revealed an irregular and hypoechoic mass (*arrow*). Microphotograph shows granulomatous mastitis (*inset*).

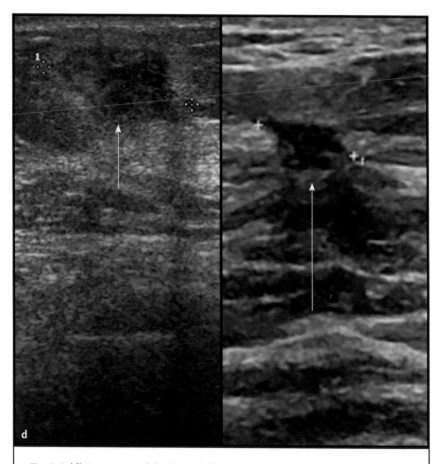

**Fig. 1.4 (d)** Comparison slide shows challenges of sonography. Idiopathic granuloma-tous mastitis (image on the left, *short arrow*) and invasive lobular adenocarcinoma (image on the right, *long arrow*). Please note that both lesions have shared imaging features, and are irregular in shape and heterogenous on ultrasound. It is not possible to establish the diagnosis based on imaging alone.

Spectrum of differential diagnoses is broad and includes malignancy, infective mastitis, tuberculous mastitis or, less frequently, Granulomatosis with polyangiitis (formerly called Wegener's granulomatosis) and foreign body reaction (**Fig. 1.4e–h**).

Please note that both malignancy and its mimics in the setting of presented mastitis may have shared imaging features.

There is skin thickening and associated increased density of the affected breast with regard to all presented entities (**Fig. 1.4i–k**).

Surgical open biopsy and repeat core biopsies carry a risk of nonhealing ulcers and sinus tract formation and should therefore be avoided in suspected cases.

## Silicone-Induced Foreign Body Granulomatous Mastitis

It is a complication of cosmetic breast augmentation. Liquid silicone may result in granulomas formation and subsequent fibrosis. This can have variable appearances on breast imaging and mimics inflammatory breast cancer. Mammography can demonstrate skin thickening with increased density throughout the breast (**Fig. 1.4e**). Sonography reveals increased echogenicity of the affected breast or silicone granulomas (**Fig. 1.4f–g**). Snowstorm appearance may also be observed. This is a very rare complication which may require mastectomy with breast reconstruction. Although injectable silicone has been proven to be unsafe, it is still utilized in many developing countries as a cheaper alternative to polymer shell implants.

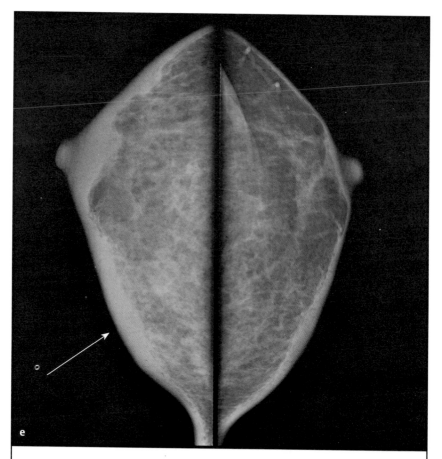

**Fig. 1.4 (e)** A 36-year-old female with a history of silicone injection for breast augmentation presented with palpably hard breast masses. Bilateral mammography revealed skin thickening and increased density throughout both breasts (*arrow*). Histology revealed foreign body granulomas formation, secondary to silicone injections. This was a complication of liquid silicone injections and subsequent foreign body reaction.

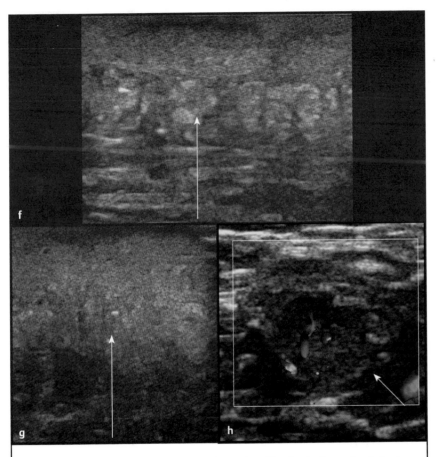

**Fig. 1.4 (f–h)** Granulomatous mastitis in the setting of foreign body reaction following silicone injections. The same patient as in **Fig. 1.4e**. High-resolution ultrasound revealed highly echogenic pattern (*long arrows*) with multiple tiny hypoechoic and ill-defined lesions. There were associated reactive lymph nodes (*short arrow*).

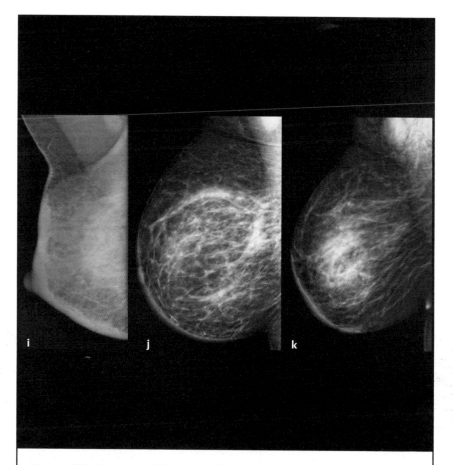

**Fig. 1.4 (i–k)** Comparison slide shows challenges of mammography. **(i)** Granulomatous mastitis in the setting of foreign body reaction, **(j)** diffuse B cell lymphoma of the breast, **(k)** and inflammatory breast cancer, namely invasive adenocarcinoma. Please note the skin thickening and associated increased density in **(i)** silicone induced mastitis which closely resembles **(j)** diffuse B cell lymphoma and **(k)** invasive adenocarcinoma.

# Parasitic Infestation of the Breast

It is a rare cause of a symptomatic breast lump. We illustrate an example of mammary filariasis.

Filariasis of the breast is mainly caused by Wuchereria bancrofti or Brugia malayi and transmitted by mosquitoes in endemic areas, predominantly tropics and subtropics of the Asian and African subcontinent.

This condition is usually unilateral and more commonly involves the upper outer quadrant of the breast. Larvae of the parasites enter and damage lymphatic vessels, which results in lymphangitis and formation of complex cystic masses (**Fig. 1.5a, b**; *arrows*). Subsequent reactive changes, and peau d'orange appearance of the affected breast mimics malignancy on physical or radiological examination (**Fig. 1.5c**).

Mammary infestation is treated with antiparasitic medication. This can be diagnosed via ultrasound-guided biopsy or blood smear by microscopic examination. Blood should be collected at night as per nocturnal periodicity of microfilariae.

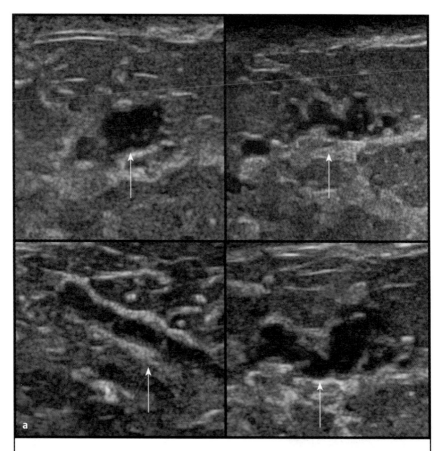

**Fig. 1.5 (a)** A 33-year-old female patient from a tropical/subtropical region was referred with a 4-month history of a firm and painless left breast mass. Physical examination raised suspicion of malignancy. Subsequent ultrasound examination revealed multiple irregular complex lesions with fluid-like components and hyperechoic contents (*arrows*). Also, see **Fig. 1.5b**. Moreover, real-time scan showed movement of some linear structures within these lesions. This was suggestive of "filarial dance sign."

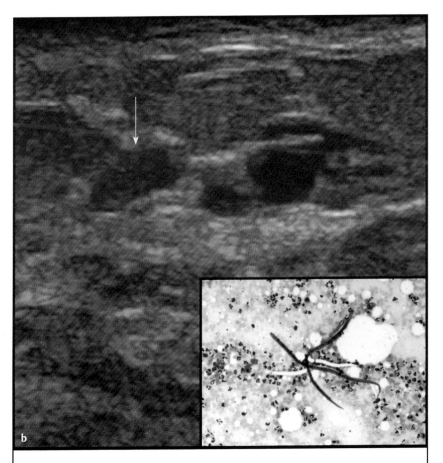

**Fig. 1.5 (b)** The same patient as in **Fig. 1.5a**. Ultrasound demonstrates an irregular complex mass with both solid-appearing and fluid-like components (*arrow*). Ultrasound-guided fine needle aspiration cytology (FNAC) revealed an adult nematode (*inset photomicrograph*).

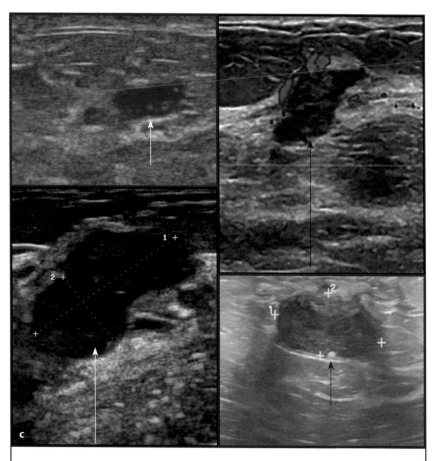

**Fig. 1.5 (c)** Comparison slide demonstrates various complex masses in the setting of malignancy and its mimics. The presented lesions consist of both solid-appearing and fluid-like components. Filariasis (*short white arrow*), mammary tuberculosis (*long white arrow*), intracystic papillary breast cancer (*long black arrow*), and idiopathic granulomatous mastitis (*short black arrow*).

# Infective Mastitis

It is commonly seen during breast feeding, as a result of nipple damage or associated with smoking and diabetes. Affected breast may be harder and painful on physical examination. The most important potential differential diagnosis is inflammatory breast carcinoma.

Infective mastitis can result in skin thickening and increased breast density on mammography.

(Refer to examples of malignancy that mimic mastitis in **Fig. 1.4j, Fig. 1.4k,** and **Fig. 1.6a**). Ultrasound can demonstrate skin thickening, ill-defined hypoechoic areas within the breast, and associated reactive axillary lymphadenopathy (**Fig. 1.6b, c**). Infection can be managed with antibiotics. However, infective mastitis can sometimes result in abscess formation and require drainage.

The resemblance between developing breast abscesses and cancers can sometimes be uncanny on ultrasound (**Fig. 1.6d, e**).

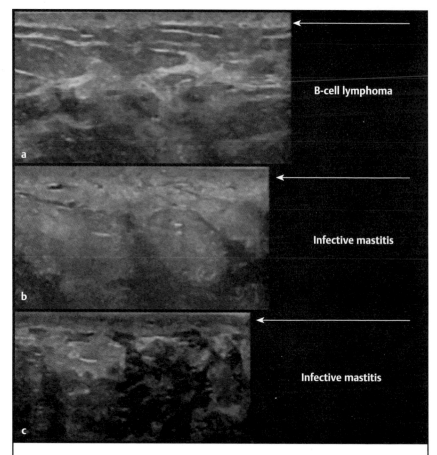

**Fig. 1.6 (a–c)** Comparison slide demonstrates challenges of sonography. **(a)** shows diffuse B cell lymphoma of the breast, which is the same patient as on **Fig. 1.4j**. **(b, c)** Demonstrate infective mastitis in a 35-year-old breast feeding female. Please note that there are skin thickening and ill-defined hypoechoic areas on all images. Inflammatory carcinoma and B cell lymphoma are important differentials and share imaging appearances.

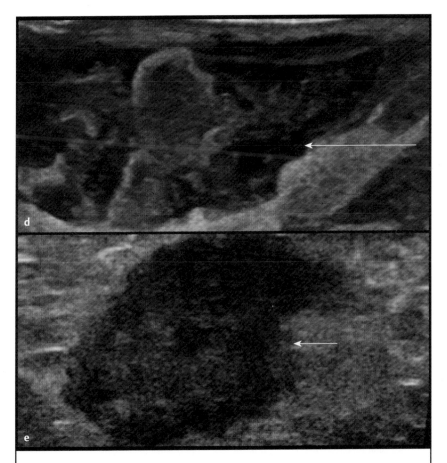

**Fig. 1.6 (d, e)** Common pitfalls on sonography—abscess versus breast malignancy. **(d)** Top image demonstrates an abscess in a 43-year-old female with a palpable painful lump. **(e)** Bottom image shows invasive ductal carcinoma of no special type in a 37-year old patient with a history of palpable left breast mass. Please note that both malignancy and its mimics have irregular margins and similar spectrum of imaging features.

## Points to Ponder

*Inflammatory and infectious diseases may mimic malignancy and create diagnostic dilemma. Therefore, a proper history and a complete clinical picture should be kept in mind while dealing with such cases.*

*Even armed with knowledge, it can be challenging to diagnose these conditions based on imaging alone. Thus, pathology and microscopic examination is often essential in establishing the final diagnosis.*

# Bibliography

Chapparia P, Singh C, Mathur N, Sharoff L. Case 12724 Filariasis in breast - Realtime US for solving this clinical dilemma. Eurorad Radiological Case Database; https://www.eurorad.org/case/12724

Chen TH. Silicone injection granulomas of the breast: treatment by subcutaneous mastectomy and immediate subpectoral breast implant. Br J Plast Surg 1995;48(2):71–76

Ikeda DM, Miyake KK. Breast Imaging: The Requisites. 3rd ed. St Louis, MO: Elsevier; 2017

Kopans DB. Breast imaging. 3rd ed. Hagerstwon, MD: Lippincott Williams & Wilkins; 2007

Pluguez-Turull CW, Nanyes JE, Quintero CJ, et al. Idiopathic granulomatous mastitis: manifestations at multimodality imaging and pitfalls. Radiographics 2018;38(2): 330–356

Shah BA, Mandawa SR. Breast Imaging A Core Review. 2nd ed. Philadelphia, PA: Wolters Kluwer; 2017

Spratt JD, Salkowski LR, Loukas M, et al. Weir & Abrahams' Imaging Atlas of Human Anatomy. 5th ed. Elsevier; 2016

Wegner U, Balschat S, Decker T, et al. Imaging findings of rare benign breast lesions: a pictorial review. Electronic Poster ECR; 2019

## Summary MCQs

### ■ Questions

Please choose true or false. More than one answer option may be correct.

*Question 1:* Which of the following statements regarding the presented cases are correct?

a) Tuberculous mastitis and idiopathic granulomatous mastitis may mimic malignancy.

b) Inflammatory and infectious diseases can present as a breast mass.

c) Mammary tuberculosis is a common manifestation of extrapulmonary localization of the disease.

d) Mammary filariasis is common entity in Western populations.

e) The exact cause of idiopathic granulomatous mastitis (IGM) is unknown.

*Question 2:* What is the first line of treatment for mammary tuberculosis?

a) Corticosteroid therapy.

b) Surgery.

c) Antituberculous treatment.

d) This is a self-limiting process and no treatment required.

e) Antiviral medication.

*Question 3:* Which of the following conditions could raise suspicion of tuberculous mastitis?

a) Recurrent breast abscesses with poor response to standard antibiotic therapy.

b) Atypical breast mass in the presence of human immunodeficiency syndrome (HIV).

c) Infectious mastitis and history of pulmonary tuberculosis.

d) Nontender breast mass and long history of diabetes.

e) Young female with autoimmune disease and nontender breast mass.

**Question 4:** Which statements with regard to the presented lymphatic filariasis of the breast are correct?

a) Parasitic infections involving the breast are common in Europe and United States.

b) Treatment consists of antiparasitic drugs.

c) Filariasis is a parasitic disease caused by nematodes and spread by mosquitoes.

d) Lymphatic filariasis can mimic malignancy on examination.

e) This is a self-limiting disease and no treatment is required.

**Question 5:** Surveillance scan of the patient with the known idiopathic granulomatous mastitis is shown in the following figure. How would you describe the sonographic findings?

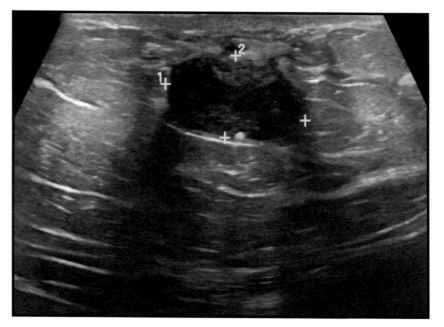

a) Complex mass with both solid-appearing and fluid-like components.

b) Simple cyst.

c) Solid ovoid mass.

d) Cyst with calcifications.

e) None of the above.

*Question 6:* Ultrasound scans of four female patients with palpable breast masses are shown in the following figure. Which statements with regard to the presented sonographic lesions are true?

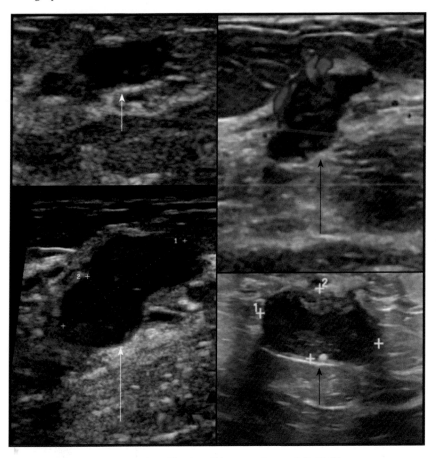

a) Presented lesions consist of both solid-appearing and fluid-like components.

b) Presented lesions have some shared imaging features.

c) Presented lesions most likely represent simple cysts.

d) All lesions represent drainable inflammatory collections.

e) Presented lesions most likely represent typical fibroadenomas.

*Question 7:* How would you describe the sonographic findings seen in the following figure?

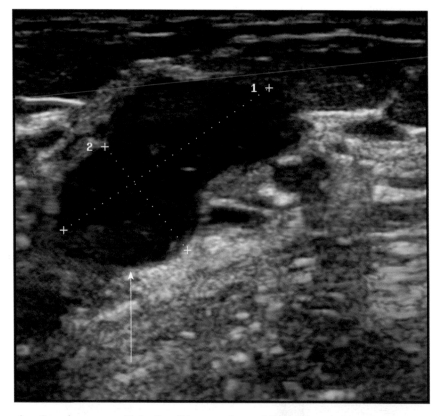

a) Complex mass with both solid-appearing and fluid-like components.

b) Simple cyst.

c) Solid ovoid mass.

d) Cyst with calcifications.

e) None of the above.

*Question 8:* What are the differential diagnoses regarding breast lesions with both solid- and fluid-appearing components?

a) Simple cyst.

b) Malignant breast lesion.

c) Complex collection resulting from infection.

d) Lipoma.

e) Intramammary lymph node.

*Question 9:* Which shape in the following figure indicates abnormality? Please choose one option.

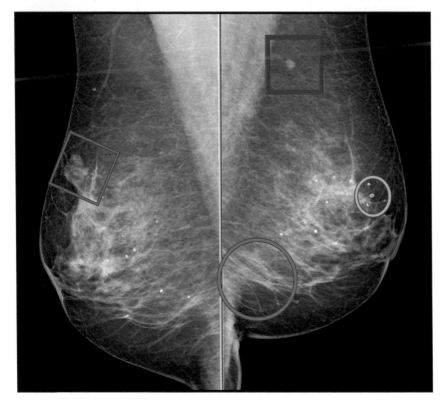

a) Yellow circle.

b) Green circle.

c) Red square.

d) Blue square.

**Question 10:** Sarcoidosis of the left breast is shown. Please match anatomic structures with correct *arrows* in the following figure.

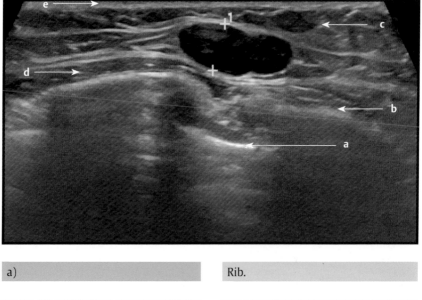

a)                              Rib.

b)                              Skin.

c)                              Pleura.

d)                              Mammary layer.

e)                              Pectoralis muscle.

# ■ Answers

*Answer 1:*

a) (T) Both tuberculous mastitis and idiopathic granulomatous mastitis conditions can present as complex breast masses indistinguishable from carcinoma. Also, see **Fig. 1.1c**, **Fig. 1.2d**, and **Fig. 1.4d.**

b) (T) Inflammatory and infectious diseases can present as complex breast masses indistinguishable from carcinoma. Also, see **Fig. 1.1c**, **Fig. 1.2d**, and **Fig. 1.4d.**

c) (F) Mammary tuberculosis is a very rare manifestation of tuberculosis.

d) (F) Mammary filariasis is endemic in the Asian and African subcontinents.

e) (T) The cause of idiopathic granulomatous mastitis remains unproven. The diagnosis is usually established by means of exclusion.

## References

Kopans DB. Breast imaging. 3rd ed. Hagerstwon, MD: Lippincott Williams & Wilkins; 2007

Pluguez-Turull CW, Nanyes JE, Quintero CJ, et al. Idiopathic granulomatous mastitis: manifestations at multimodality imaging and pitfalls. Radiographics 2018;38(2): 330–356

*Answer 2:*

a) (F) Corticosteroid therapy is contraindicated in case of tuberculosis as it may cause disease progression.

b) (F) Surgery may be considered in case of poor response to treatment and extensive, symptomatic disease.

c) (T) Antituberculous treatment is the first line of treatment and targeted long-term antibiotic therapy is required.

d) (F) This is not a self-limiting process. Tuberculous mastitis requires targeted pharmacotherapy.

e) (F) Antiviral medication is not indicated as this condition is not caused by a virus. Tuberculous mastitis is a bacterial infection caused by *Mycobacterium tuberculosis.*

# References

Kopans DB. Breast imaging. 3rd ed. Hagerstwon, MD: Lippincott Williams & Wilkins; 2007

Pluguez-Turull CW, Nanyes JE, Quintero CJ, et al. Idiopathic granulomatous mastitis: manifestations at multimodality imaging and pitfalls. Radiographics 2018;38(2): 330–356

*Answer 3:*

a) (T) Tuberculosis will not respond to standard antibiotic therapy, thus, recurrent breast abscesses with poor response to antibiotics may raise suspicion of tuberculous mastitis.

b) (T) Immunodeficiency increases the risk of mammary tuberculosis, especially in high-risk populations and in endemic areas.

c) (T) Tuberculous mastitis can be seen in high-risk populations, persons with pulmonary tuberculosis, or in endemic areas.

d) (F) Nontender breast mass and long history of diabetes could raise the suspicion of diabetic mastopathy in the setting of long-standing diabetes. Tuberculous mastitis predisposes to breast abscess formation.

e) (F) Young female with autoimmune disease and nontender breast mass could raise the suspicion of lymphocytic mastopathy in the setting of autoimmune disease. Tuberculous mastitis predisposes to breast abscess formation.

# Reference

Kopans DB. Breast imaging. 3rd ed. Hagerstwon, MD: Lippincott Williams & Wilkins; 2007

*Answer 4:*

a) (F) Parasitic infections are endemic in tropics and subtropics.

b) (T) Filariasis can be effectively treated with antiparasitics.

c) (T) Filariasis is caused by Wuchereria bancrofti which affects lymphatic channels. In addition, this disease is spread by mosquitoes.

d) (T) Lymphatic filariasis can mimic malignancy on physical examination and present as a complex cystic mass on sonography.

e) (F) Filariasis requires treatment with antiparasitic medication.

# References

Chapparia P, Singh C, Mathur N, Sharoff L. Case 12724 Filariasis in breast - Realtime US for solving this clinical dilemma. Eurorad Radiological Case Database; https://www.eurorad.org/case/12724

Kopans DB. Breast imaging. 3rd ed. Hagerstwon, MD: Lippincott Williams & Wilkins; 2007

Wegner U, Balschat S, Decker T, et al. Imaging findings of rare benign breast lesions: a pictorial review. Electronic Poster ECR; 2019

*Answer 5:*

a) (T) The sonogram demonstrates a complex mass with both hyperechoic solid-appearing (See **Fig. 1.2c**, *short arrows*) and fluid-like components more centrally (See **Fig. 1.2c**, *long arrows*).

b) (F) Simple cyst should be anechoic without solid, hyperechoic components.

c) (F) This mass is irregular in shape and consists of both solid and fluid-appearing components.

d) (F) No cyst with calcifications identified.

e) (F) The first option is correct, as there is a solitary complex and irregular mass.

# Reference

Kopans DB. Breast imaging. 3rd ed. Hagerstwon, MD: Lippincott Williams & Wilkins; 2007

*Answer 6:*

a) (T) The lesion presents as complex masses with both solid-appearing and fluid-like components (see **Fig. 1.1d**).

b) (T) These masses are different in shape. However, all lesions present as complex masses with both solid-appearing and fluid-like components (See explanation in **Fig. 1.1d** solid-appearing components [*short arrow*] and fluid-like component more centrally [*long arrow*]).

c) (F) Simple cysts do not have solid-appearing components.

d) (F) These are complex lesions which contain solid-appearing, hyperechoic components.

e) (F) Typical fibroadenoma does not contain fluid-like components.

# References

Chapparia P, Singh C, Mathur N, Sharoff L. Case 12724 Filariasis in breast - Realtime US for solving this clinical dilemma. Eurorad Radiological Case Database; https://www.eurorad.org/case/12724

Ikeda DM, Miyake KK. Breast Imaging: The Requisites. 3rd ed. St Louis, MO: Elsevier; 2017

Kopans DB. Breast imaging. 3rd ed. Hagerstwon, MD: Lippincott Williams & Wilkins; 2007

Pluguez-Turull CW, Nanyes JE, Quintero CJ, et al. Idiopathic Granulomatous Mastitis: Manifestations at Multimodality Imaging and Pitfalls. Radiographics 2018;38(2): 330–356

Wegner U, Balschat S, Decker T, et al. Imaging Findings of Rare Benign Breast Lesions: A Pictorial Review. Electronic Poster ECR; 2019

## Answer 7:

a)  (T) The sonogram demonstrates a complex mass with both hyperechoic solid-appearing (See **Fig. 1.1d**, *short arrows*) and anechoic fluid-like components more centrally (See **Fig. 1.1d**, *long arrow*).

b)  (F) It is not a cyst. Simple cysts are anechoic without solid, hyperechoic components.

c)  (F) This mass is irregular in shape and consists of both solid- and fluid-appearing components.

d)  (F) No cyst with calcifications identified.

e)  (F) The first option is correct, as there is a solitary complex and irregular mass.

# Reference

Kopans DB. Breast imaging. 3rd ed. Hagerstwon, MD: Lippincott Williams & Wilkins; 2007

## Answer 8:

a)  (F) Simple cyst does not have solid-appearing components.

b)  (T) Various malignant lesions have both solid-appearing and fluid-like components, for example, intracystic papillary carcinoma (**Fig. 1.1c**, *short arrow*), thus, such complex masses warrant microscopic examination.

c) (T) Collection resulting from inflammatory and infectious diseases of the breast may present as complex masses, with both solid-appearing and fluid-like components (**Fig. 1.2b**, *short arrow*).

d) (F) A lipoma is regular in shape and does not contain any fluid-appearing components

e) (F) A typical lymph node does not contain any fluid-like components.

## Reference

Kopans DB. Breast imaging. 3rd ed. Hagerstwon, MD: Lippincott Williams & Wilkins; 2007

*Answer 9:*

a) (F) Yellow circle indicates oil cysts.

b) (F) Green circle indicates breast tissue.

c) (F) Red square indicates lymph node.

d) (T) Blue square indicates mammographic abnormality with irregular margins.

*Answer 10:*

| | |
|---|---|
| a) | Pleura. |
| b) | Rib. |
| c) | Mammary layer. |
| d) | Pectoralis muscle. |
| e) | Skin. |

## Reference

Spratt JD, Salkowski LR, Loukas M, et al. Weir & Abrahams' Imaging Atlas of Human Anatomy. 5th ed. Elsevier; 2016

# Chapter 2

# Metabolic and Immunologic Conditions

# Metabolic and Immunologic Conditions

## Learning Objectives:

1. To highlight immunologic and metabolic conditions that may simulate malignant process with regard to breast imaging and physical examination.
2. To discuss associated histopathology and management of patients.
3. To gather and strengthen valuable knowledge during the course of a comprehensive quiz with feedback and diagnostic pearls.

## Introduction

There are limited immunologic or metabolic conditions which may result in a breast mass formation and give rise to misleading appearances on imaging.

Both Type 1 and Type 2 diabetes have been explored along their dimensions but their manifestations in breast imaging have not been given the due explicit significance they deserve until it manifests as a mass-forming pathology which confuses the diagnostics team with regard to malignancy. The feature of relapsing disease again puts a doubt in the minds of even well-experienced radiologists.

We will illustrate various malignancy mimics in the setting of chronic diabetes, lymphocytic mastopathy and mammary sarcoidosis, which may create dilemma in appropriate diagnosis, causing patient apprehension and worry.

# Diabetic Mastopathy

It is a purely benign, chronic fibroinflammatory breast disease in the setting of long-standing diabetes mellitus type 1 or 2.

Clinical presentation of a large painless firm breast mass in male or female patient may create a worrisome scenario for the patient, warranting aggressive treatment due to the fear possibility of neoplasm and lack of awareness of this presentation of diabetes.

Several medical descriptors such as diabetic mastopathy, lymphocytic mastopathy, or sclerosing lymphocytic lobulitis may be used by various authors, as they represent the same spectrum of histopathological features.

Namely, this condition is characterized by perivascular lymphocytic infiltration and fibrous stromal proliferation, due to excessive glycosylation in diabetes, which results in fibrosis and subsequent palpably hard breast mass formation.

This uncommon entity is a complication of chronic impaired glucose metabolism in diabetic patients (**Flowchart 2.1**). The exact etiology still remains unclear; however, it is believed to be human leukocyte antigen (HLA)-associated autoimmune process.

Imaging findings on sonography and mammography may be concerning for a breast carcinoma.

Associated fibrosis as a sequel to long-standing or poorly controlled disease may lead to distortion on mammography (**Fig. 2.1**, *arrow*). This process results in palpable, hypoechoic, and poorly-defined masses formation on ultrasound (**Fig. 2.2**, **Fig. 2.3**, and **Fig. 2.4**). Sonographic appearances often resemble "flammable" hypoechoic pattern (**Fig. 2.5** and **Fig. 2.6a–d**).

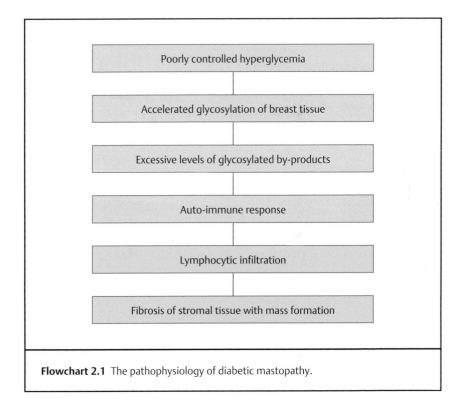

**Flowchart 2.1** The pathophysiology of diabetic mastopathy.

Interestingly, sonographically evident, small volume disease with posterior acoustic shadowing can be even more misleading and indistinguishable from malignancy (**Fig. 2.6a**).

This condition is entirely benign and requires no surgical treatment. However, biopsy is highly recommended in cases of doubtful diagnosis to reassure our patients. The patients should also be made aware of the recurrence of the disease on background of diabetes even after requested surgical excision.

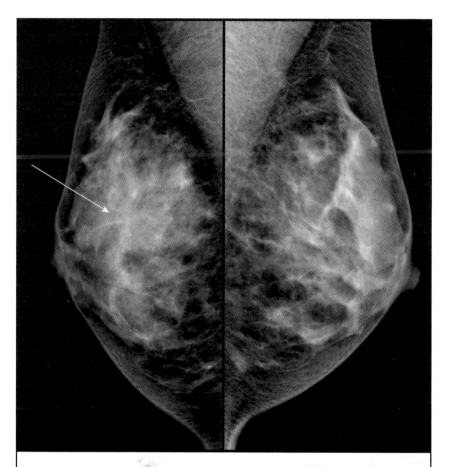

**Fig. 2.1** A 34-year old female with a long-standing diabetes type 1 presented with a palpable right upper breast mass. Right MLO view shows distortion (*arrow*) in the setting of resultant fibrosis. Abbreviation: MLO, mediolateral oblique view.

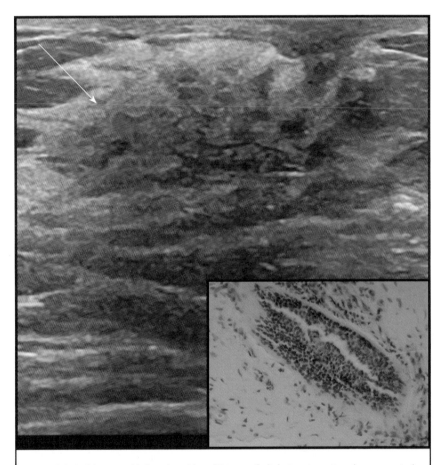

**Fig. 2.2** A 28-year old female with a history of diabetes type 1, who presented with right retroareolar firm lump. Ultrasound revealed poorly-defined distortion of decreased echogenicity, forming a "flammable pattern" (*arrow*). Mammography was not performed. This is correlated with a palpably hard area. Pathology showed dominant lymphocytic aggregates in periductal distribution (*inset*).

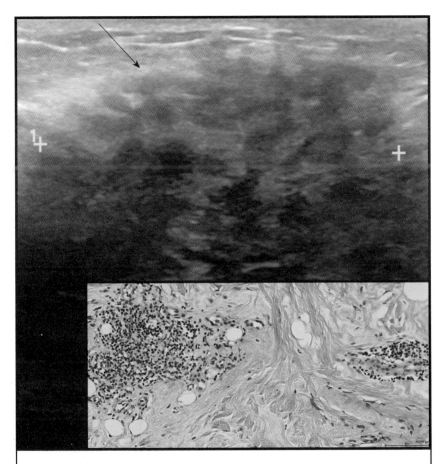

**Fig. 2.3** Example of a similar sonographic pattern; however, regarding a more advanced disease. A 30-year old patient with 25-year history of diabetes type 1. Palpably hard mass at 12 o'clock corresponds to an ill-defined shadowing mass (*arrow*). Mammography was not performed. Associated microphotograph (*inset*).

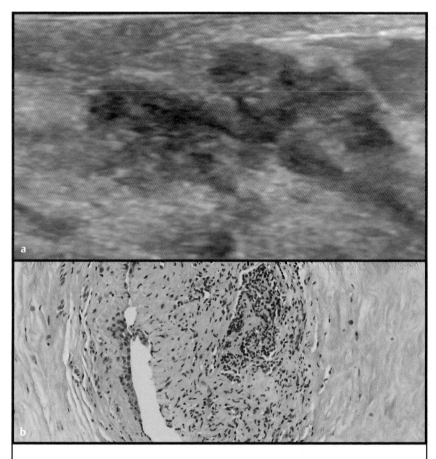

**Fig. 2.4** A 46-year old diabetic patient with a palpable mass near the nipple was referred to the breast unit. **(a)** Ultrasound showed poorly-defined "flammable" pattern of decreased echogenicity. This was mammographically occult. **(b)** Associated microphotograph showed diabetic mastopathy.

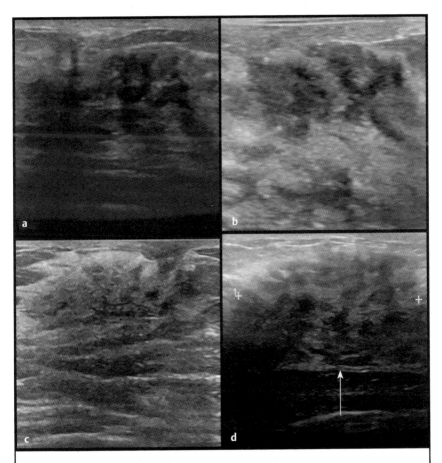

**Fig. 2.5** Comparison slide shows imaging patterns in the setting of long-standing diabetes type 1 in four different patients. Please note that all patients (**a–d**) presented with palpably hard masses. Moreover, advanced diabetic mastopathy associated with **d** (*arrow*) presented as suspicious distortion on mammography (also see **Fig. 2.1**).

## Evolution and Progression of Diabetic Mastopathy

Diabetic mastopathy on imaging may begin as a focal hypoechoic mass with ill-defined margins and distal acoustic shadowing. (**Fig. 2.6a**).

As the disease progresses, a number of such focal areas as well as the size of the mass may progress and can be easier to diagnose than the early stage of disease. Advanced stadium may present as a more diffuse process with resultant extensive fibrosis and progressive palpable abnormality (**Fig. 2.6b**).

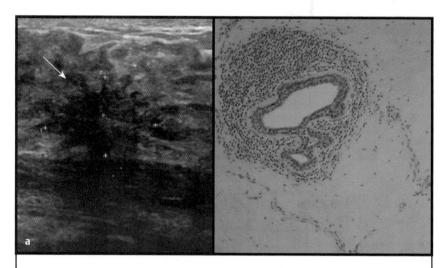

**Fig. 2.6 (a)** A 30-year old patient with a history of long-standing diabetes type 1 presented with a left retroareolar lump. Sonography revealed ill-defined area mimicking carcinoma (*arrow*). Biopsy confirmed benign changes in the setting of diabetic mastopathy (microphotograph on the right shows lymphocytic infiltrates).

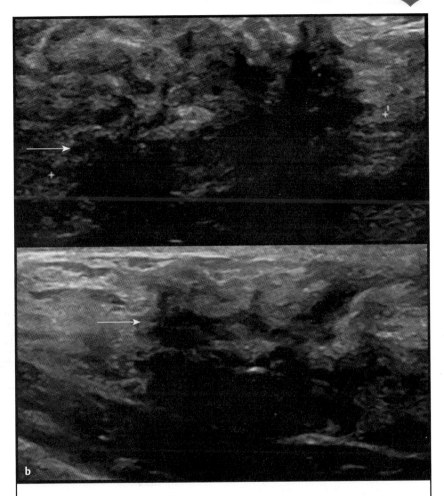

**Fig. 2.6 (b)** The same patient represented 1 year later, and the affected symptomatic area has increased in size as well as another focal lesion appeared adjacent to the index lesion (*short arrows*). Biopsies again confirmed changes in the setting of chronic diabetes.

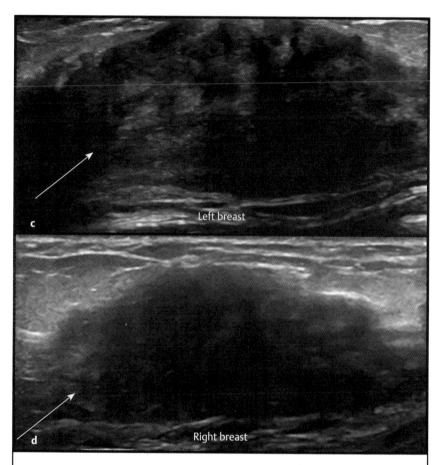

**Fig. 2.6 (c, d)** This is a different patient than on **Fig. 2.6a, b**. However, both medical history and clinical presentation are similar. A 30-year old female with a history of poorly-controlled and long-standing diabetes type 1, presented with bilateral retro areolar lumps. Ultrasound of both breasts is shown (*arrows*). Sonography showed bilateral, centrally located hypoechoic masses in keeping with palpable abnormalities. Histology confirmed benign changes in the setting of patient's diabetic mastopathy.

# Lymphocytic Mastitis

Clinical and imaging manifestations similar to diabetes can also be related to several autoimmune diseases like systemic lupus erythematosus, autoimmune thyroiditis, or rheumatoid arthritis, secondary to even pregnancy.

The age of presentation is pre and perimenopausal, which is similar to malignancies. The patient may have unilateral as well as bilateral disease with multiple nontender nodules.

There is an increased amount of growth factors leading to deposition of collagen which, in turn, leads to scarring and mass formation.

Mammography may show an area of distortion, representing the background scarring, secondary to the autoimmune response and inflammatory change (**Fig. 2.7a**, *arrow*).

Serial mammograms may either show gradual resolution or unchanged appearance of disease often posttreatment; however, during the initial imaging, subtle progression of the disease process may be seen.

Chronic cases may show multiple foci of scattered calcifications– usually monomorphic, resulting from the sequel of vasculitis in associated immunological diseases.

Involvement of skin is usually seen in systemic lupus erythematosus with discreet scattered calcifications and subcutaneous nodules all over the body and may hint toward the diagnosis.

On subsequent imaging, ultrasound may show focal hypoechoic homogenous mass with varying degrees of posterior acoustic shadowing (**Fig. 2.7b, c**).

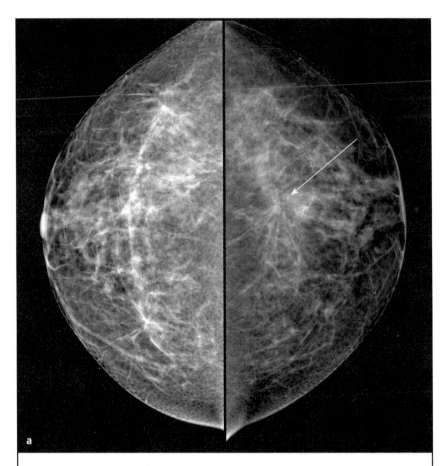

**Fig. 2.7 (a)** A 37-year old breast-feeding female with a 3-month history of a palpable breast lump. Mammography revealed distortion in the central left breast (please see left CC view, *arrow*). Histology showed lymphocytic mastopathy. This patient did not have diabetes and the exact cause was unknown. However, it is suggested that nonspecific factors during pregnancy regulate immune system and may influence autoimmune processes. Abbreviation: CC, craniocaudal.

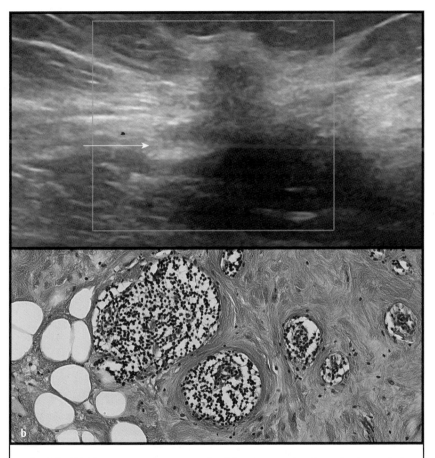

**Fig. 2.7 (b)** The same patient as on **Fig. 2.7a**. Sonography showed a hypoechoic mass which was taller than wide (*arrow*). Breast malignancy was suspected. However, histology showed lymphocytic mastopathy/sclerosing lymphocytic lobulitis (*bottom image*).

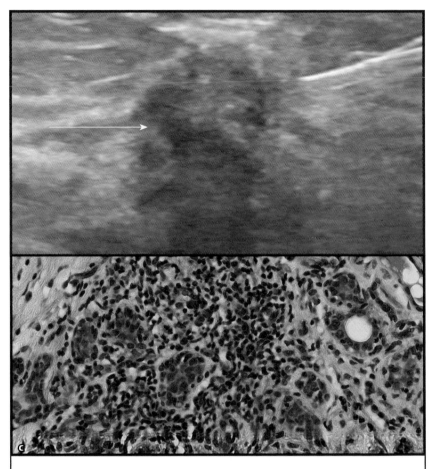

**Fig. 2.7** **(c)** A 27-year old female patient presented with a palpable nodularity in the upper outer quadrant of the right breast. Ultrasound showed hypoechoic mass (*arrow*). Histopathology revealed lymphocytic sclerosing lobulitis/lymphocytic mastopathy (*bottom image*) Diabetes was excluded during subsequent biochemical studies. The cause of the lymphocytic infiltrates in the breast remained unknown.

# Sarcoidosis

It is another interesting medical condition that often mimics metastatic disease. This is a multisystemic and immune-mediated granulomatous disease.

Sarcoid can affect any organ; more commonly, it involves lungs, lymphatic system, or the skin. Manifestation in the breast is very rare and can present as a palpable mass due to sarcoid granulomas formation. Patients may also present as a primary breast mass in the absence of systemic manifestation which may be confused for metastatic disease (**Fig. 2.8c**).

Unlike previously discussed cases of granulomatous mastitis, sarcoidosis is not associated with significant inflammatory changes, complex masses with fluid-like components, or chronic breast abscesses.

Sonography can demonstrate hypoechoic, well-defined, or irregular lesions which can be confused with breast malignancy or metastatic lymph nodes (**Fig. 2.8a** and **Fig. 2.8c**).

Fine needle aspiration is recommended and histology shows noncaseating granulomas with epitheliod cells (**Fig. 2.8b**). Concurrent high-levels of serum ACE (angiotensin-converting enzyme) establish the diagnosis.

Compared with other granulomatous pathologies, sarcoid breast lesions are more rounded and show smooth margins (**Fig. 2.8c**). Another interesting manifestation of mammary sarcoidosis is associated with formation of numerous hypoechoic nodules throughout the affected breast and skin (**Fig. 2.9**).

Mammary sarcoidosis can be diagnosed via core needle biopsy and microscopic examination.

In some cases of symptomatic and extensive multisystemic disease, medications that suppress immune system may be considered. Surgical treatment of mammary sarcoidosis is not necessary. This is benign granulomatous disease that can be managed conservatively.

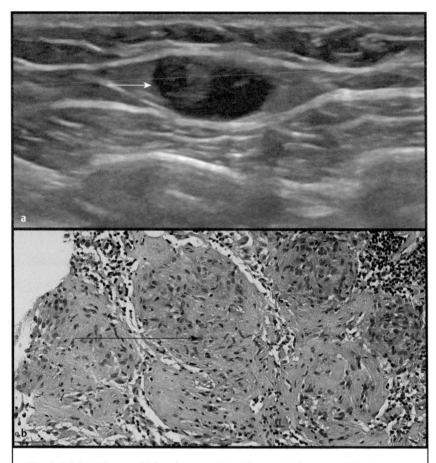

**Fig. 2.8 (a)** A 36-year old female presented with a palpable mass within the outer left breast. Ultrasound showed a well-defined hypoechoic lesion (*short white arrow*). **(b)** Microphotograph showing multiple small noncaseating granulomas (*long black arrow*).

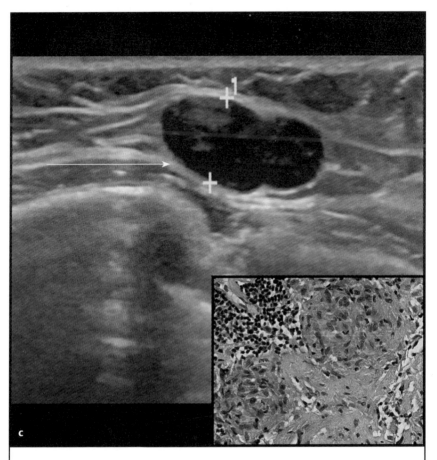

**Fig. 2.8 (c)** The same patient as on **Fig. 2.8a, b**. Hypoechoic mass mimicking pathological lymph node on sonography *arrow*). Microphotograph shows simple epithelioid granulomas (*inset*).

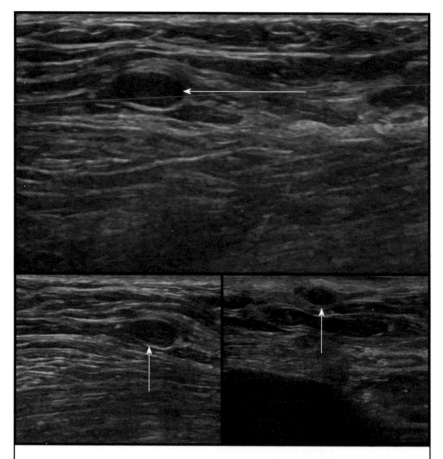

**Fig. 2.9** A 63-year old female with a history of long-standing sarcoidosis presented with new palpable lumps within the right breast. Ultrasound was performed for verification as it was essential to exclude any potential malignant process. This showed multiple hypoechoic nodules of various size and location, some of them were more superficial and palpable (*arrows*). Multiple core biopsies were performed, and subsequent histology confirmed granulomas in the setting of patient's main disease.

# Bibliography

D'Orsi CJ, Sickles EA, Ellen B; American College of Radiology. ACR BI-RADS Atlas der Mammadiagnostik. Berlin, Germany: Springer; 2016

Ikeda DM, Miyake KK. Breast Imaging: The Requisites. 3rd ed. St Louis, MO: Elsevier; 2017

Kopans DB. Breast imaging. 3rd ed. Hagerstwon, MD: Lippincott Williams & Wilkins; 2007

Mak CW, Chou CK, Chen SY, Lee PS, Chang JM. Case report: diabetic mastopathy. Br J Radiol 2003;76(903):192–194

Piccinni MP, Lombardelli L, Logiodice F, Kullolli O, Parronchi P, Romagnani S. How pregnancy can affect autoimmune diseases progression? Clin Mol Allergy 2016;14:11

Pluguez-Turull CW, Nanyes JE, Quintero CJ, et al. Idiopathic granulomatous mastitis: manifestations at multimodality imaging and pitfalls. Radiographics 2018;38(2): 330–356

Shah BA, Mandawa SR. Breast Imaging A Core Review. 2nd ed. Philadelphia, PA: Wolters Kluwer; 2017

Spratt JD, Salkowski LR, Loukas M, et al. Weir & Abrahams' Imaging Atlas of Human Anatomy. 5th ed. Elsevier; 2016

Tabar L, Dean PB. Teaching Atlas of Mammography. 4th ed. Thieme; 2011

Taylor K, Britton P, O'Keeffe S, Wallis MG. Quantification of the UK 5-point breast imaging classification and mapping to BI-RADS to facilitate comparison with international literature. Br J Radiol 2011;84(1007):1005–1010

Wegner U, Balschat S, Decker T, et al. Imaging Findings of Rare Benign Breast Lesions: A Pictorial Review. Electronic Poster ECR; 2019

## Summary MCQs

### ■ Questions

Please choose true or false. More than one option may be correct.

*Question 1:* Which of the following statements regarding the presented cases are correct?

a) Hashimoto thyroiditis and diabetes type 1 are associated with lymphocytic mastopathy.

b) Mammary sarcoidosis is very common and can mimic malignancy on imaging.

c) Diabetic mastopathy carries risk of malignant transformation and requires surgery.

d) Diabetic mastopathy or lymphocytic mastopathy represents the same spectrum of histopathological features.

e) Lymphocytic mastopathy is a benign condition which does not require surgery.

*Question 2:* Diabetic mastopathy is shown. Please match anatomy structures with correct *arrows*.

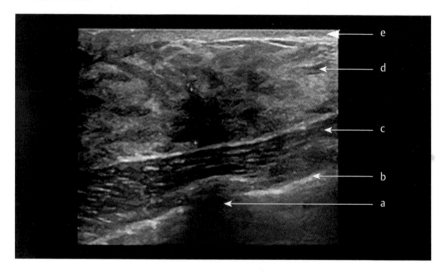

| a) | Rib. |
| b) | Skin. |
| c) | Pleura. |
| d) | Mammary layer. |
| e) | Pectoralis muscle. |

***Question 3:*** Lymphocytic mastopathy is shown. How would you describe mammographic findings?

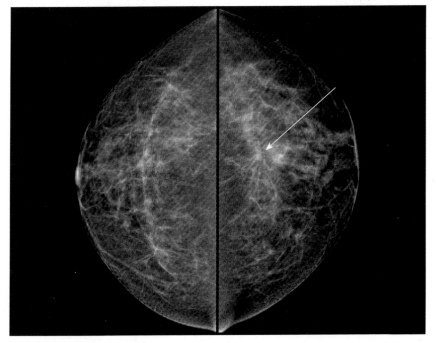

a) Architectural distortion.

b) No significant findings identified and suspected pathology is occult.

c) Suspicious microcalcifications.

d) High-density circular/oval lesion.

e) Low-density circular/oval lesion.

**Question 4:** Mammary sarcoidosis is shown. How would you describe the sonographic findings?

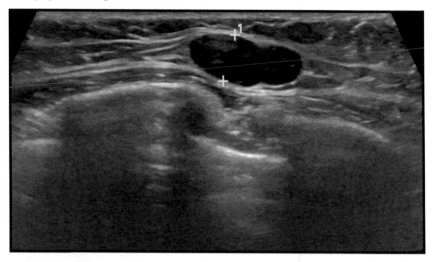

a)  Anechoic round lesion.

b)  Hyperechoic round subcutaneous lesion.

c)  A well-defined hypoechoic lesion.

d)  An irregular hypoechoic lesion.

e)  Normal.

**Question 5:** What is the preferred diagnostic modality in case of a palpable lump in a young woman with diabetes type 1 and Hashimoto thyroiditis?

a)  Mammography.

b)  Breast magnetic resonance imaging (MRI).

c)  Digital breast tomosynthesis (DBT.)

d)  Breast ultrasound.

e)  Contrast-enhanced mammography (CESM).

**Question 6:** Ultrasound of a symptomatic diabetic patient is shown. What is the preferred next diagnostic step?

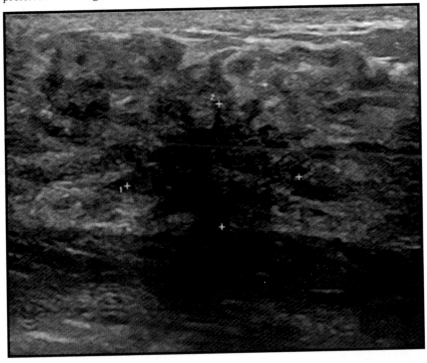

a)   No further management required.

b)   Ultrasound-guided core needle biopsy.

c)   Breast MRI.

d)   Stereotactic biopsy.

e)   Aspiration.

**Question 7:** Which conditions may increase the risk of developing lymphocytic mastopathy?

a)   Lymphoma.

b)   Autoimmune thyroid disease.

c)   Diabetes.

d)   Sarcoidosis.

e)   Human immunodeficiency virus (HIV) coinfection.

*Question 8:* Given the final benign diagnosis of diabetic mastopathy, what is the appropriate breast imaging reporting and database system score (BI-RADS) assessment?

a)  BI-RADS 5.

b)  BI-RADS 1.

c)  BI-RADS 2.

d)  BI-RADS 4.

*Question 9:* Diabetic mastopathy is shown. Which shape indicates abnormality?

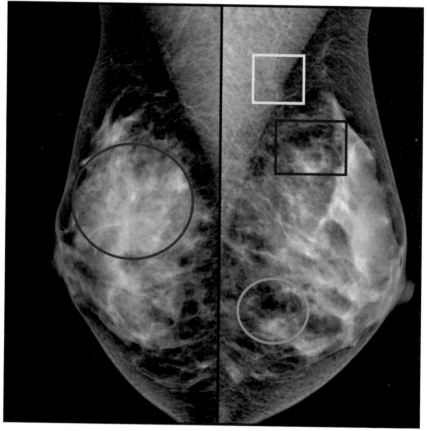

a)  Yellow square.

b)  Green circle.

c)  Red circle.

d)  Blue square.

**Question 10:** In sonography, which of the following features may be suggestive of malignancy?

a) Irregular.

b) Smooth margins.

c) Taller than wide.

d) Ill-defined.

e) Well-defined.

**Question 11:** Which of the conditions below may present as breast nodules and subcutaneous nodules? More than one option may be correct.

a) Lymphocytic mastopathy in the setting of Hashimoto thyroiditis.

b) Mammary sarcoidosis.

c) Diabetic mastopathy.

d) Lymphocytic mastopathy in the setting of systemic lupus erythematosus.

e) Pregnancy-associated immune mastopathy.

# ■ Answers

*Answer 1:*

a) (T) Lymphocytic mastopathy is associated with diabetes and autoimmune diseases.

b) (F) Sarcoidosis of the breast is extremely rare. However, this condition may present as a palpable hypoechoic irregular mass. This can mimic both pathological lymph node or carcinoma.

c) (F) Diabetic mastopathy is purely benign and no invasive surgical procedures are required.

d) (T) Namely, diabetic mastopathy or lymphocytic mastopathy condition is characterized by perivascular lymphocytic infiltration and fibrous stromal proliferation which subsequently results in fibrous palpably hard breast mass formation.

e) (T) Lymphocytic mastopathy is a benign condition and no treatment is required.

## Reference

Kopans DB. Breast imaging. 3rd ed. Hagerstwon, MD: Lippincott Williams & Wilkins; 2007

Pluguez-Turull CW, Nanyes JE, Quintero CJ, et al. Idiopathic granulomatous mastitis: manifestations at multimodality imaging and pitfalls. Radiographics 2018;38(2): 330–356

Shah BA, Mandawa SR. Breast Imaging A Core Review. 2nd ed. Philadelphia, PA: Wolters Kluwer; 2017

*Answer 2:*

| | |
|---|---|
| a) | Rib. |
| b) | Pleura. |
| c) | Pectoralis muscle. |
| d) | Mammary layer. |
| e) | Skin. |

## Reference

Spratt JD, Salkowski LR, Loukas M, et al. Weir & Abrahams' Imaging Atlas of Human Anatomy. 5th ed. Elsevier; 2016

*Answer 3:*

a) (T) Architectural distortion with spicules in the form of radiating structure is identified.

b) (F) Architectural distortion is noted and suspected pathology is not mammographically occult.

c) (F) No calcifications are identified.

d) (F) This lesion has a different imaging pattern and no definite mass is visualized. Architectural distortion seen.

e) (F) This lesion has a different imaging pattern and no overt mass is visualized. Architectural distortion seen.

# Reference

Tabar L, Dean PB. Teaching Atlas of Mammography. 4th ed. Thieme; 2011

*Answer 4:*

a)  (F) This is neither anechoic nor round in shape.

b)  (F) Hyperechoic, round, and subcutaneous lesions are the features of a typical lipoma.

c)  (T) This is a well-defined and hypoechoic lesion; also, this is elongated and oval in shape and all the margins are well-visualized. Imaging features are suggestive of an abnormal lymph node.

d)  (F) The sonographic mass is well-defined and regular in shape.

e)  (F) A well-defined hypoechoic mass is identified.

# Reference

Kopans DB. Breast imaging. 3rd ed. Hagerstwon, MD: Lippincott Williams & Wilkins; 2007

*Answer 5:*

a)  (F) This patient can be examined with an ultrasound and without additional radiation doses received during mammography.

b)  (F) Palpable breast lump in a young woman is an indication for an ultrasound.

c)  (F) The patient can be examined with an ultrasound and without additional radiation doses received during DBT.

d)  (T) Palpable mass in a young woman can be easily assessed with an ultrasound.

e)  (F) The patient can be easily examined with an ultrasound and without additional radiation doses received during contrast-enhanced mammography.

# Reference

Shah BA, Mandawa SR. Breast Imaging A Core Review. 2nd ed. Philadelphia, PA: Wolters Kluwer; 2017

*Answer 6:*

a)  (F) Biopsy is required to exclude malignancy.

b)  (T) An irregular and hypoechoic lesion is visualized. Ultrasound-guided core needle biopsy is the preferred next diagnostic step as microscopic verification is needed to establish the final diagnosis.

c)  (F) A solitary mass on ultrasound is not an indication for MRI.

d)  (F) Stereotactic biopsy could be an option with regard to a mammographic abnormality.

e)  (F) This is a solid mass. No fluid to aspirate identified.

## References

Kopans DB. Breast imaging. 3rd ed. Hagerstwon, MD: Lippincott Williams & Wilkins; 2007

Shah BA, Mandawa SR. Breast Imaging A Core Review. 2nd ed. Philadelphia, PA: Wolters Kluwer; 2017

*Answer 7:*

a)  (F) Lymphocytic mastopathy is associated with diabetes and autoimmune diseases.

b)  (T) Lymphocytic mastopathy is associated with diabetes and autoimmune diseases.

c)  (T) Lymphocytic mastopathy is associated with diabetes and autoimmune diseases.

d)  (F) Lymphocytic mastopathy is associated with diabetes and autoimmune diseases. There is no association with sarcoidosis.

e)  (F) Lymphocytic mastopathy is associated with diabetes and autoimmune diseases. There is no connection with HIV virus.

## References

Kopans DB. Breast imaging. 3rd ed. Hagerstwon, MD: Lippincott Williams & Wilkins; 2007

Shah BA, Mandawa SR. Breast Imaging A Core Review. 2nd ed. Philadelphia, PA: Wolters Kluwer; 2017

*Answer 8:*

a)  (F) BI-RADS 5 category means highly suspicious of malignancy.

b)  (F) BI-RADS 1 category is consistent with a normal result.

c)  (T) BI-RADS 2 category means benign findings.

d)  (F) BI-RADS 4 category is reserved for lesions that are not typical of malignancy but are sufficiently suspicious and require biopsy.

# References

D'Orsi CJ, Sickles EA, Ellen B; American College of Radiology. ACR BI-RADS Atlas der Mammadiagnostik. Berlin, Germany: Springer; 2016

Kopans DB. Breast imaging. 3rd ed. Hagerstwon, MD: Lippincott Williams & Wilkins; 2007

Shah BA, Mandawa SR. Breast Imaging A Core Review. 2nd ed. Philadelphia, PA: Wolters Kluwer; 2017

*Answer 9:*

a)  (F) Yellow square demonstrates normal left axillary tail.

b)  (F) Green circle shows unremarkable dense breast tissue.

c)  (T) Red circle reveals distortion. Please note spicules and radiating structure within the circle in the following figure (*arrow*).

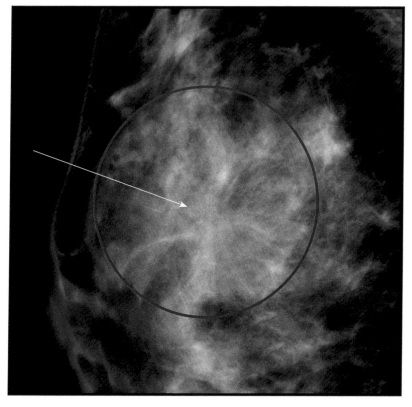

d)  (F) Blue square shows normal breast tissue. No mammographic abnormality identified.

## Reference

Tabar L, Dean PB. Teaching Atlas of Mammography. 4th ed. Thieme; 2011

*Answer 10:*

a) (T) Irregular shape raises suspicion of malignancy.

b) (F) Smooth margins do not add to our level of suspicion and are often associated with benign lesions.

c) (T) Taller than wide growth pattern should be considered suspicious on ultrasound. Biopsy is necessary to exclude malignancy.

d) (T) Ill-defined or poorly-defined lesions are concerning for malignant process.

e) (F) Well-defined feature does not increase our level of suspicion and is often related to benign lesions.

## References

Georgian-Smith D, Lawton T. Breast Imaging and Pathologic Correlations: A Pattern-Based Approach. Philadelphia, PA: Wolters Kluwer; 2014

Kopans DB. Breast imaging. 3rd ed. Hagerstwon, MD: Lippincott Williams & Wilkins; 2007

*Answer 11:*

a) (F) Only breast and thyroid pseudo-nodules can be seen in lymphocytic mastopathy in the setting of Hashimoto thyroiditis.

b) (T) Both breast nodules and subcutaneous nodules can be seen in sarcoidosis.

c) (F) Only breast nodules are seen in diabetic mastopathy.

d) (T) Breast as well as subcutaneous nodules can be seen in lymphocytic mastopathy associated with systemic lupus erythematosus.

e) (F) Only breast nodules are seen in pregnancy-associated immune mastopathy. Skin nodules are not associated with this entity.

## References

Georgian-Smith D, Lawton T. Breast Imaging and Pathologic Correlations: A Pattern-Based Approach. Philadelphia, PA: Wolters Kluwer; 2014

Sabaté JM, Clotet M, Gómez A, De Las Heras P, Torrubia S, Salinas T. Radiologic evaluation of uncommon inflammatory and reactive breast disorders. Radiographics 2005;25(2): 411–424

# Chapter 3

## Lesions of Vascular and Neural Origin

# Chapter 3

# Lesions of Vascular and Neural Origin

## Learning Objectives:

1. To aid adequate imaging including doppler for excluding benign etiologies which may appear worrisome.

2. To discuss diagnostic pathway and further management of the affected patients.

3. To empower quick recapitulation of the topic content through a quiz-based approach.

## Introduction

This is the third part of the series that will strengthen your expertise in recognition and management of potential malignancy mimics.

This module illustrates a very unique collection from international sources and will familiarize you with the most challenging conditions of vascular and neural origin.

The main goal is to inspire you to turn your new knowledge into action.

## Vascular Lesions

Vascular lesions of breast can be classified into benign and malignant, but in our chapter we shall be emphasizing on the benign counterparts. They represent a very rare diagnostic dilemma in breast radiology and may mislead dedicated breast imagers regardless of experience.

We will discuss interesting cases of mammary angiomatosis, vascular malformation, and breast aneurysm or hemangioma that simulate cancer.

## Mammary Angiomatosis

This is one of the rarest vascular tumors in breast radiology. They clinically present as gradually progressive breast lump.

Appearances on sonography and mammography may be a matter of concern for primary malignancy.

Mammography may show well-defined homogeneous opacity with irregular margins and increased density (**Fig. 3.1a**, *arrows*).

Sonographic features of a heterogeneously hyper to hypoechoic, often a diffuse mass with irregular margins, may raise concerns for malignancy such as lobular breast carcinoma (**Fig. 3.1b, c**). Physical examination can reveal nontender and palpable mass.

This unusual condition carries the risk of local recurrence. Thus, wide local excision with clear margins is required. Mastectomy can be considered in case of a very extensive disease.

This is an entirely benign entity and prognosis is excellent. To the best of knowledge there is no proven association between mammary angiomatosis and von Hippel-Lindau disease or other phakomatoses.

Specimen histology usually show large irregular spaces lined by flattened endothelial cells lacking muscular wall. Sometimes, red blood cells can be seen in these spaces.

The main differential diagnosis includes angiosarcoma and carcinoma of the breast.

Moreover, breast aneurysms, hemangiomas, or various vascular malformations may have misleading appearances on imaging (**Fig. 3.2** and **Fig. 3.3**).

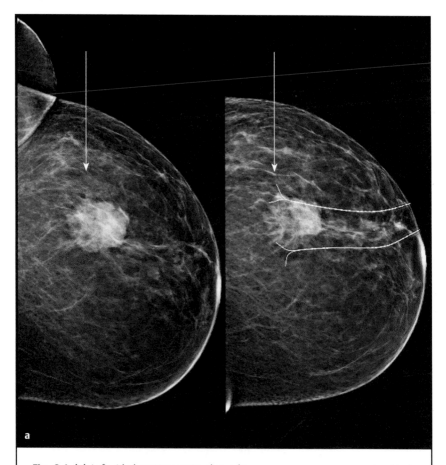

**Fig. 3.1 (a)** Left-sided mammogram shows biopsy-proven mammary angiomatosis (*arrows*). Moreover, the image on the right shows wire localization prior to wide local excision. (Right image) Wire localization can be used to guide breast surgeons and helps with regard to adequate, complete removal of the mass. This presents as a lobulated and low-density mass. Physical examination revealed palpable and nontender abnormality.

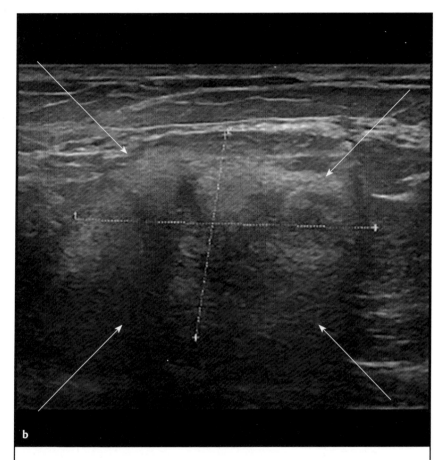

**Fig. 3.1 (b)** The same patient as in **Fig. 3.1a**. Ultrasound revealed an ill-defined, heterogenous and irregular mass (*arrows*). Please see explanations on **Fig. 3.1c**.

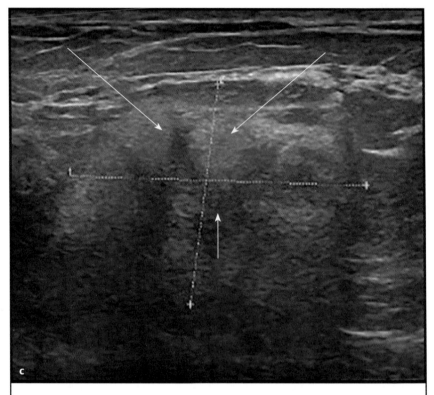

**Fig. 3.1 (c)** The same patient as in **Fig. 3.1a, b**. Mammary angiomatosis on ultrasound. The presented mass is irregular in shape and heterogenous. It contains hyperechoic components peripherally (*long arrows*) and hypoechoic component centrally (*short arrow*).

# Thrombosed Pseudoaneurysm

We illustrate this interesting example of a thrombosed pseudoaneurysm (**Fig. 3.2a, b**).

They may present as mildly pulsatile, growing breast lump. Mammography can show smooth mixed-density oval to round opacity, often with adjacent overlap of vessels (**Fig. 3.2a**).

On sonography, a hypo to anechoic oval breast mass with distal acoustic enhancement was correlated. Color Doppler showed turbulent flow within the mass and a few twigs of radiating vessels from the mass. (**Fig. 3.2c**)

True aneurysms of breast are rarely encountered and need to be differentiated from breast carcinoma (**Fig. 3.2d**, *long arrow* and **Fig. 3.2e**, *short arrow*) or angiosarcoma.

## Mammary Hemangioma

Breast hemangiomas are superficial oval or lobulated masses, often nonpalpable due to soft consistency, and can be broadly described as capillary or cavernous, depending on the dimensions of cystic spaces within the mass. Patients are asymptomatic and these lesions are often detected on screening mammograms.

On mammography, the density may be similar to the fibroglandular component (**Fig. 3.3a, b**). In addition, there may be variable degree of calcification.

On sonography, the masses are oval or lobulated and oriented parallel; however, the internal echotexture of the hemangioma can sometimes mimic a complex cystic malignancy (**Fig. 3.3c**).

Color Doppler therefore becomes essential in the evaluation of cystic or pulsatile masses where intralesional flow can be detected and spectral Doppler can characterize the pattern of flow—arterial in cases of hemangioma (**Fig. 3.3d**).

These lesions are often biopsied in cases where malignancy is suspected but profuse bleeding postbiopsy may hint toward the diagnosis. Histology of the biopsy samples may show dilated tubular channels filled with red blood cells.

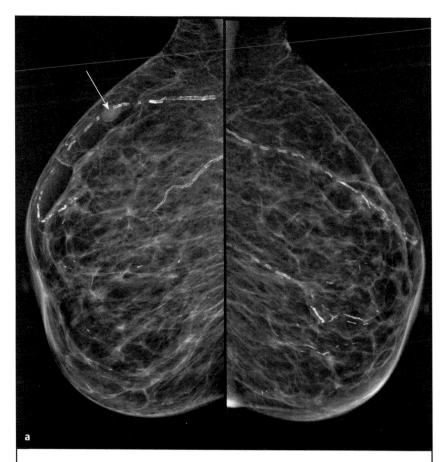

**Fig. 3.2 (a)** An 81-year-old symptomatic female presented with a palpable mass within the upper outer quadrant of the right breast. Bilateral mammography showed a subcentimeter mass (*arrow*).

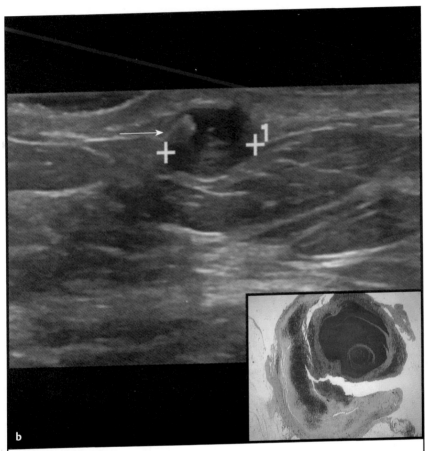

**Fig. 3.2 (b)** The same patient as on **Fig. 3.2a**. Ultrasound shows a hypoechoic lesion with hyperechoic intraluminal thrombus (*arrow*). Microphotograph confirms a benign vascular lesion (*inset*).

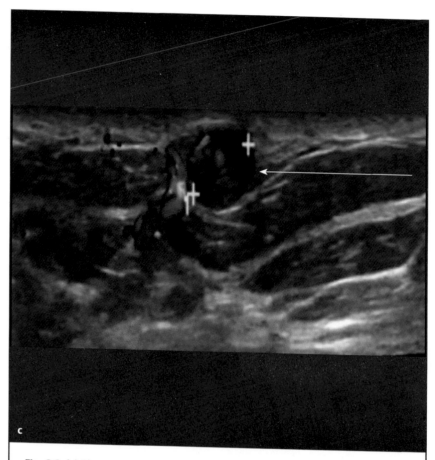

**Fig. 3.2 (c)** The same patient as in **Fig. 3.2a, b**. Color Doppler confirms a vascular lesion with distal acoustic enhancement (*arrow*) confirming the benign vascular origin of the lesion.

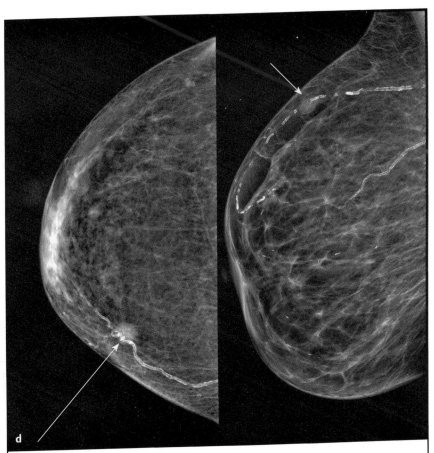

**Fig. 3.2 (d)** Comparison slide shows challenges of mammography. Invasive ductal carcinoma of no special type (*long arrow*) and a partially thrombosed aneurysm (*short arrow*). Carcinoma has slightly spiculated margins in contrast to a smoothly marginated aneurysm. However, please note that this is not obvious on mammography, and it is not possible to establish the diagnosis based on imaging alone.

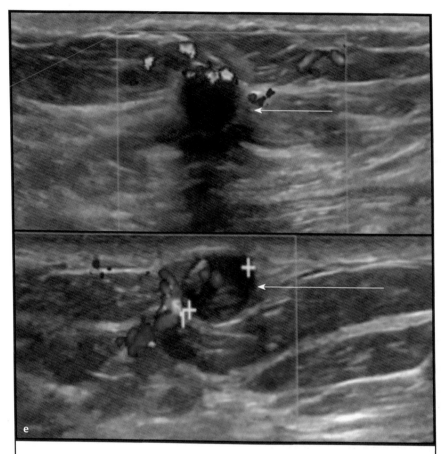

**Fig. 3.2 (e)** Comparison slide shows challenges on ultrasonography. The same patients as on **Fig. 3.2d**. The top image shows invasive ductal carcinoma of no special type (*short arrow*). The bottom image shows a thrombosed aneurysm (*long arrow*). Carcinoma demonstrates posterior acoustic shadowing which is absent in case of the presented benign aneurysm.

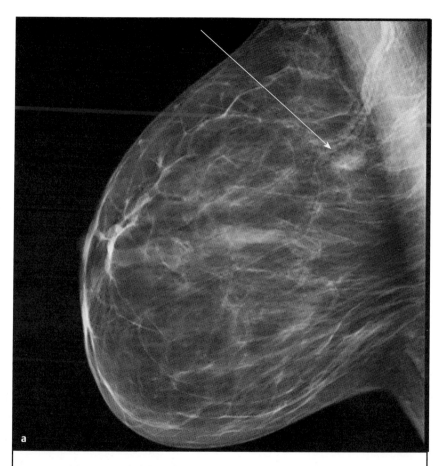

**Fig. 3.3 (a)** A 59-year old female was recalled from screening. Right MLO view showed an ill-defined and low-density mass (*arrow*). It was a painless, nonpalpable mass. Abbreviation: MLO, mediolateral oblique.

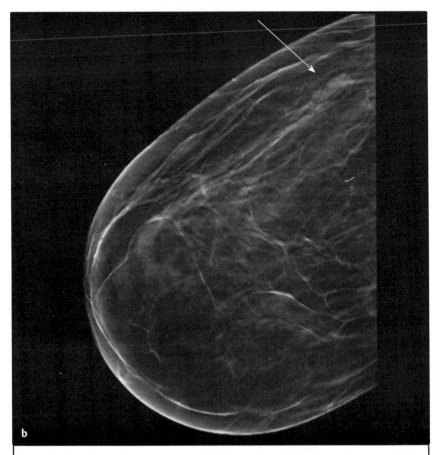

**Fig. 3.3 (b)** The same patient as in **Fig. 3.3a**. Right breast tomosynthesis showed a solitary low-density lesion within the upper outer quadrant (*long arrow*).

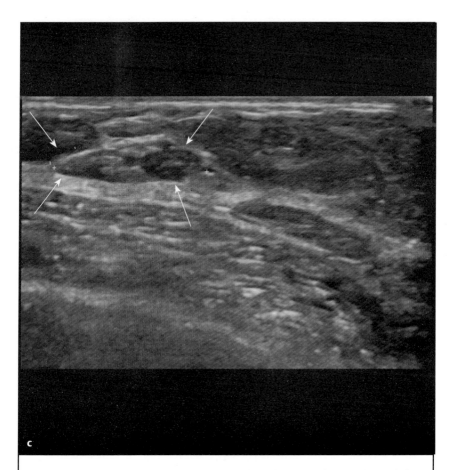

c

**Fig. 3.3 (c)** The same patient as in **Fig. 3.3a, b**. Right breast ultrasound revealed a benign vascular malformation. This demonstrated high flow on Doppler. However, the lesion comprised both arterial and compressible venous elements.

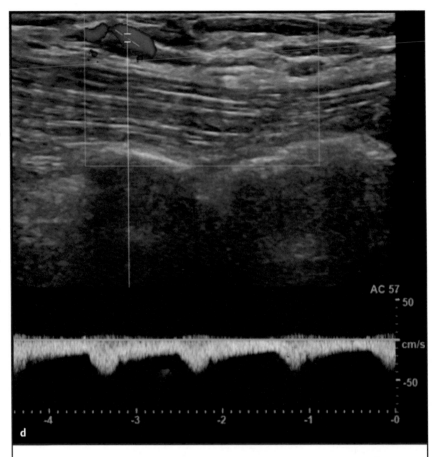

**Fig. 3.3 (d)** The same patient as in **Fig. 3.3a–c**. The lesion demonstrated arterial flow on Doppler.

# Lesions of Neural Origin

Lesions of neural origin in the breast are very uncommon. We illustrate granular cell tumor of the breast, and a case of neurofibromatosis type 1 with associated cutaneous neurofibromas.

## Granular Cell Tumor (GCT)

It is a benign tumor with malignant clinical and imaging characteristics. Patients commonly present with rapidly growing lump which is often tender. This mass originates from Schwann cells and can present as a palpably firm mass on physical examination. Often associated coexistence of prominent axillary lymph nodes may raise the suspicion of locally advanced disease with metastasis. Enlarged lymph nodes can be usually due to inflammatory change or purely coincidental.

Mammography can show an indistinctly defined oval to round mass with irregular margins. Ultrasound shows hypo to anechoic mass with fuzzy margins.

Imaging features may be indistinguishable from those of a carcinoma and biopsy needs to be performed to exclude a malignant process (**Fig. 3.4a–c**). This entity is benign, but carries a risk of local recurrence, and wide local excision with clear margins is required.

Very rare and limited malignant presentations in the setting of presumed GCT transformations have also been reported.

Histology confirms oval spindle-shaped cells and multinucleated giant cells. (**Fig. 3.4c**).

The cells are positive for CD 68 and S100, hence supporting the diagnosis.

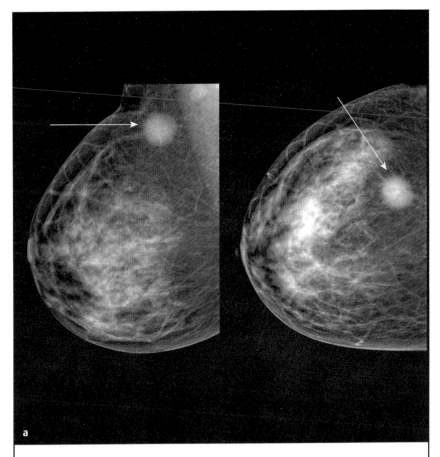

**Fig. 3.4 (a)** Right-sided mammogram, MLO view on the left, and CC view on the right. A 46-year old female presented with a palpably hard right breast mass. Mammography showed a well-defined mass within the upper outer quadrant of the right breast and close to the pectoralis muscle (*arrows*). Abbreviations: CC, craniocaudal; MLO, mediolateral oblique.

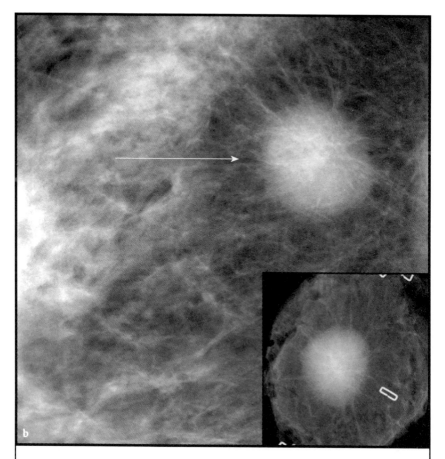

**Fig. 3.4 (b)** The same patient as in **Fig. 3.4a**. Right-sided magnification view shows a dense mass with subtle spiculations (*arrow*). Please note wide, local excision specimen with the mass in the central part (*inset*).

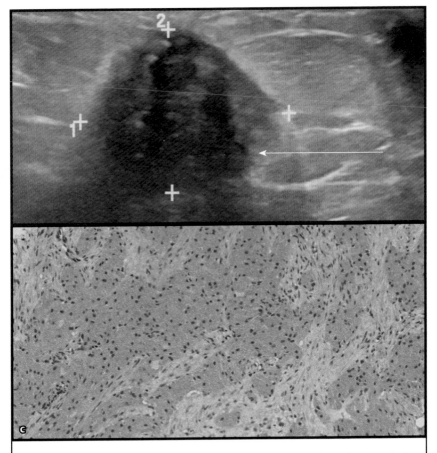

**Fig. 3.4 (c)** The same patient as seen in **Fig. 3.4a, b**. Ultrasound showed a hypoechoic and irregular mass (*arrow*). There was associated posterior acoustic shadowing. No skin thickening was observed. Microphotograph shows features of a GCT with granular cytoplasm, small central round nuclei, and small nucleoli. The cells were positive for CD 68 and S100 which supported the diagnosis. There was no evidence of malignancy or atypia such as necrosis, pleomorphism, or more mitotic figures. Abbreviation: GCT, granular cell tumor.

# Cutaneous Neurofibromas

These disorders most commonly present as multiple epidermal nodules.

These can present as palpable breast lumps on physical examination and raise our suspicion of malignancy. Moreover, it is suggested that patients with Von Recklinghausen disease have increased risk of developing a breast cancer.

We illustrate high-resolution ultrasound imaging of a male patient with NF1 who presented with a palpable right breast lump in **Fig. 3.5a, b**.

Neurofibromas are round to oval and well-defined hypoechoic lesions with benign features on sonography (**Fig. 3.5a, b**).

Cutaneous neurofibromas are benign tumors and do not require any surgical treatment, unless they grow large or cause cosmetic problems.

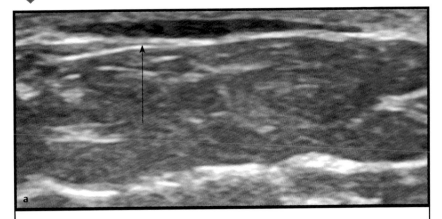

**Fig. 3.5 (a)** A 27-year-old male patient with a history of neurofibromatosis type 1 was referred to the symptomatic breast unit with a palpable lump within the upper inner right breast. Ultrasound revealed multiple well-defined, flat, and hypoechoic cutaneous lesions in both breasts (*arrow*). Imaging features were entirely benign in keeping with cutaneous neurofibromas. There were no associated suspicious features. Changes in the setting of the patient's main disease were more prominent on the right side.

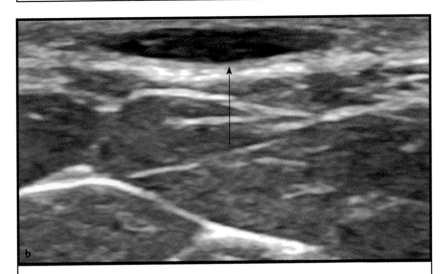

**Fig. 3.5 (b)** The same patient as in **Fig. 3.5a**. There were similar benign-appearing cutaneous lesions within the contralateral left breast (*arrow*). These represented multiple neurofibromas in the setting of the patient's known Von Recklinghausen disease.

## Points to Ponder

*Lesions of vascular and neural origin can mimic carcinoma.*

*However, these are very "rare zebras" in breast radiology and it is essential to exclude malignancy at first instance.*

*"When you hear hoof beats, think of horses not zebras."*

—Dr. Theodore Woodward

# Bibliography

Bruce R. Korf. The phakomatoses. Clin Dermatol 2005; (Jan-Feb):78–84

Chen J, Wang L, Xu J, et al. Malignant granular cell tumor with breast metastasis: a case report and review of the literature. Oncol Lett 2012;4(1):63–66

C. Romera de la Fuente, J. Echeveste Aizpurua, R. Pelaez Chato, B Rodriguez-Vigil Junco, A. Cisneros Calvo, B. Martinez de Guerenu Ortuoste, Vitoria-Gasteiz. Phakomatoses: what every radiologist should know. Educational Exhibit ECR 2014; doi:10.1594/ecr2014/C-1029

Devi Meenal Jagannathan. Benign granular- cell tumor of the breast case report and literature review. Radiol Case Rep 2015;10:1116

Gavriilidis P, Michalopoulou I, Baliaka A, Nikolaidou A. Granular cell breast tumor mimicking infiltrating carcinoma. BMJ Case Rep 2013;2013:bcr2012008178

Gogas J, Markopoulos C, Kouskos E, et al. Granular cell tumor of the breast: a rare lesion resembling breast cancer. Eur J Gynaecol Oncol 2002;23(4):333–334

Howell SJ, Hockenhull K, Gareth Evans D. Increased risk of breast cancer in neurofibromatosis type 1: current insights. Breast Cancer 2017;9:531–536

Ji J, Hemminki K. Familial blood vessel tumors and subsequent cancers. Ann Oncol 2007; (Jul):1260–1267

Khan AN, Turnbull I, Al-Okaili R. Imaging in von Hippel-Lindau Syndrome. Manchester, UK: Medscape; 2015

Kim EK, Lee MK, Oh KK. Granular cell tumor of the breast. Yonsei Med J 2000;41(5):673–675

Kopans DB. Breast imaging. 3rd ed. Hagerstwon, MD: Lippincott Williams & Wilkins; 2007

Mandava A, Ravuri PR, Konathan R. High-resolution ultrasound imaging of cutaneous lesions. Indian J Radiol Imaging 2013;23:269–277

Shah BA, Mandawa SR. Breast Imaging A Core Review. 2nd ed. Philadelphia, PA: Wolters Kluwer; 2017

Sundaram M. Angiomatosis of the breast: a rare lesion. J Clin Diagn Res 2012;6(4): 709–711

Wegner U, Balschat S, Decker T, et al. Imaging Findings of Rare Benign Breast Lesions: a Pictorial Review. Electronic Poster ECR; 2019

Wegner U, Balschat S, Decker T, Ryan AG. Rare coexistence of a cerebellar hemangio-blastoma and angiomatosis of the breast without underlying phakomatosis. J Clin Imaging Sci 2019;9(8):1–4

Wegner U, Juette A, Ryan AG, et al. Granular cell tumor (GCT) of the breast: case report of uncommon benign neural tumor with malignant imaging characteristics. J Med Clin Res & Rev. 2019;3(1):1–3

## Summary MCQs

### ■ Questions

Please choose true or false. More than one answer option may be correct.

*Question 1:* Which of the following statements regarding the presented cases are correct?

a) Mammary angiomatosis and granular cell tumor (GCT) carry the risk of local recurrence.

b) Lesions of vascular and neural origin may mimic malignancy on imaging.

c) GCT is a vascular lesion.

d) Mammary angiomatosis originates from Schwann cells.

e) Cutaneous neurofibromas have benign sonographic features.

**Question 2:** Mammary angiomatosis is shown in the following figure. How would you describe the mammographic features?

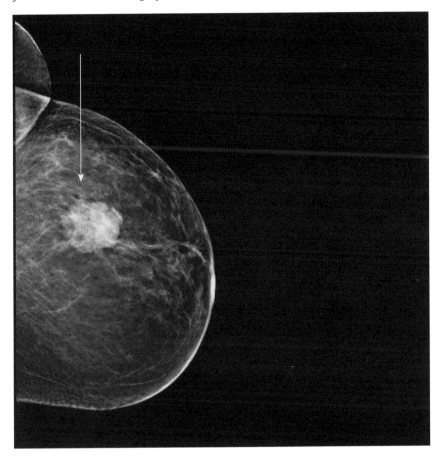

a)   Oval lesion with extensive halo sign.

b)   Architectural distortion.

c)   No significant findings identified.

d)   Microcalcifications.

e)   Irregular mass.

**Question 3:** Angiomatosis of the breast is shown in the following figure. How would you describe the sonographic features?

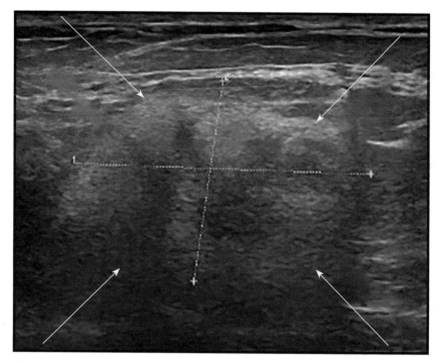

a) Anechoic round and sharply defined lesion.

b) Hyperechoic round subcutaneous lesion.

c) An ovoid well-defined hypoechoic lesion.

d) An irregular heterogenous lesion.

e) An ovoid heterogeneous lesion.

*Question 4:* Ultrasound image of a symptomatic female patient with a palpable breast mass is shown in the following figure. What would be the next diagnostic step?

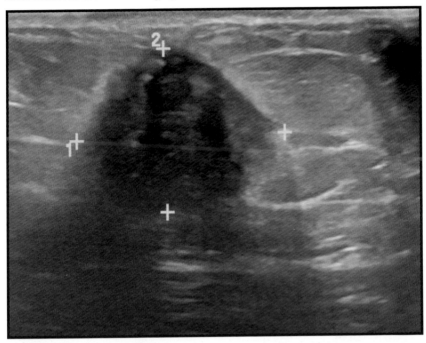

a)  No further management required.

b)  Ultrasound-guided core needle biopsy.

c)  Breast MRI.

d)  Stereotactic biopsy.

e)  Aspiration.

**Question 5:** Sonography images of a carcinoma and thrombosed aneurysm are shown in the following figure. Which image belongs to the patient with an aneurysm and why?

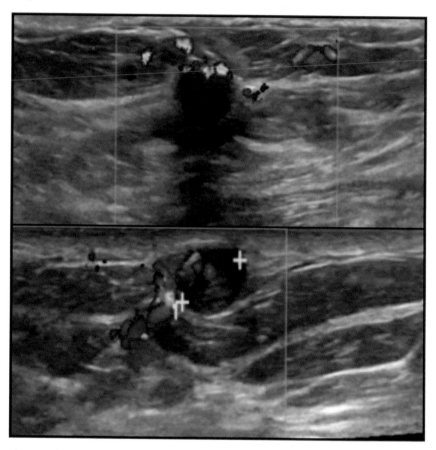

a) Top image could represent a benign vascular lesion as it shows typical benign appearances on ultrasound.

b) Top image could represent an aneurysm as the mass is taller than wide and irregular in shape, with associated posterior acoustic shadowing.

c) Bottom image does not belong to the patient due to its suspicious sonographic appearance.

d) Bottom image is related to the patient with an aneurysm as it shows a well-defined, oval mass with intralesional Doppler flow.

e) None of the above is correct.

# Answers

*Answer 1:*

a) (T) Both benign tumors carry the risk of local recurrence, thus wide local excision with clear margins is recommended.

b) (T) Lesions of vascular and neural origin may mimic malignancy on imaging as shown in the images below:

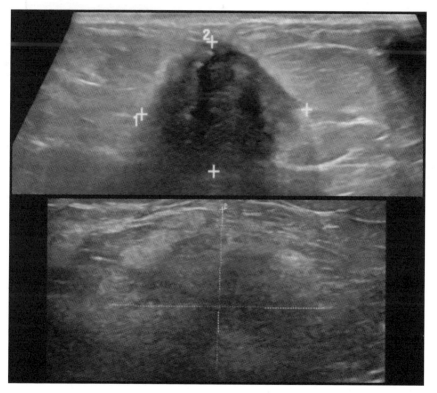

c) (F) GCT is a benign neural tumor which originates from the Schwann cells.

d) (F) Mammary angiomatosis does not originate from the Schwann cells as angiomatosis of the breast is a benign vascular tumor.

e) (T) Sonographic appearances of cutaneous neurofibromas are benign. Cutaneous neurofibromas presents as round to oval, well-defined, flat and hypoechoic cutaneous lesions, as shown in the below image (*arrow*).

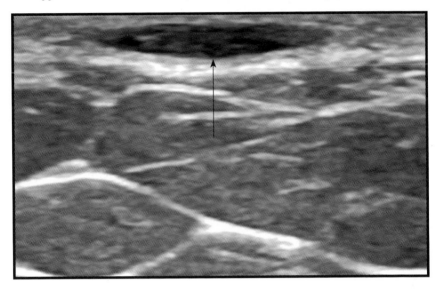

## References

Kopans DB. Breast imaging. 3rd ed. Hagerstwon, MD: Lippincott Williams & Wilkins; 2007

Tabar L, Dean PB. Teaching Atlas of Mammography. 4th ed. Thieme; 2011

*Answer 2:*

a) (F) No air outlining or halo sign seen.

b) (F) No radiating structure with spicules is visualized.

c) (F) Irregular mass identified.

d) (F) No calcification is identified.

e) (T) This mass is irregular in shape.

## Reference

Tabar L, Dean PB. Teaching Atlas of Mammography. 4th ed. Thieme; 2011

*Answer 3:*

a)   (F) These are features of a simple cyst.

b)   (F) These are features of a typical lipoma.

c)   (F) These are classical features of a fibroadenoma.

d)   (T) An irregular and heterogeneous lesion is identified. See the following figure:

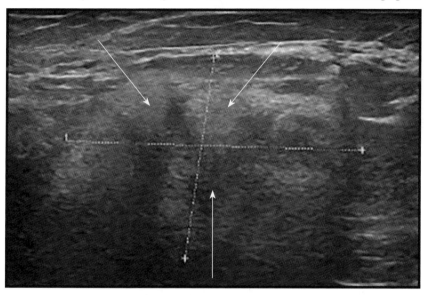

e)   (F) An irregular mass is identified which is not ovoid in shape.

## References

Kopans DB. Breast imaging. 3rd ed. Hagerstwon, MD: Lippincott Williams & Wilkins; 2007

Tabar L, Dean PB. Teaching Atlas of Mammography. 4th ed. Thieme; 2011

*Answer 4:*

a)   (F) Biopsy is required to exclude malignancy.

b)   (T) Ultrasound-guided core needle biopsy is the preferred next diagnostic step as microscopic verification is needed to establish the final diagnosis.

c)   (F) A solitary, solid mass on ultrasound is not an indication for MRI.

d)   (F) This could be an option with regard to mammographic abnormality.

e)   (F) This is a solid mass. No drainable collection identified.

# References

Kopans DB. Breast imaging. 3rd ed. Hagerstwon, MD: Lippincott Williams & Wilkins; 2007

Shah BA, Mandawa SR. Breast Imaging A Core Review. 2nd ed. Philadelphia, PA: Wolters Kluwer; 2017

*Answer 5:*

a)  (F) Top image represents malignancy as the lesion is irregular in shape and demonstrates posterior acoustic shadowing.

b)  (F) The lesion on the top image demonstrates malignant sonographic characteristics: posterior acoustic shadowing and irregular margins.

c)  (F) Bottom image does belong to the patient with an aneurysm as the lesion appears more benign and has no posterior acoustic shadowing.

d)  (T) This appears benign on imaging and shows well-circumscribed oval lesion without posterior shadowing. Intralesional flow on Doppler application correlates with the final diagnosis.

e)  (F) Option d is correct.

# Reference

Kopans DB. Breast imaging. 3rd ed. Hagerstwon, MD: Lippincott Williams & Wilkins; 2007

# Chapter 4

## Proliferative Disorders

# Proliferative Disorders

## Learning Objectives:

1. To present various proliferative conditions that can simulate breast cancer.
2. To reinforce the imaging features by correlating them with histopathology and subsequent treatment pathway.
3. Quiz-based approach for quick revision of the topics.

## Introduction

This chapter will familiarize you with various interesting, proliferative changes and other breast lesions. The emphasis is also on the type of malignancy each pattern mimics, which can provide the key for differentials for accurate diagnosis. This module of the series is designed to identify your strengths and reinforce the knowledge from the earlier parts.

## Pseudoangiomatous Hyperplasia (PASH)

This is a noncancerous and proliferative disorder of the breast. It represents benign mesenchymal overgrowth and is often seen either in premenopausal women or postmenopausal women treated with hormone replacement therapy. Hormonal influence associated with developement of pseudoangiomatous hyperplasia (PASH) is suggested.

It may clinically present as a palpable, nontender breast mass and simulate carcinoma on imaging.

Two subtypes of PASH have been described in literature– microscopic and tumoral. The microscopic type is often diagnosed in pathological specimens; however, the tumoral type is very rare, and in this chapter, we shall be focusing on the tumoral type which mimics breast cancer.

This benign lesion can also be found incidentally. The radiological features are nonspecific and may warrant histopathological verification. Most patients may have no mammographic abnormality.

However, most common findings associated with PASH are well or partially circumscribed masses without architectural distortion or microcalcification.

It can be seen as asymmetry or an island of normal glandular tissue.

Ultrasound shows hypoechoic lesions whose margins may be poorly defined or irregular in shape (**Fig. 4.1a–c**).

Histopathology shows a network of stromal spaces with "slit-like" channels (*insets* in **Fig. 4.1a–c**). No blood cells can be seen in these slit-like spaces.

Similar slit-like spaces are also seen in low-grade angiosarcoma, but ultrasound may help in differentiating such cases, as the angiosarcoma has more cystic spaces than PASH. In addition, color Doppler flow patterns are very pronounced in angiosarcoma.

Once the diagnosis of PASH is confirmed on histology, surgical excision is not recommended as this is a purely benign entity which does not increase the risk of malignancy.

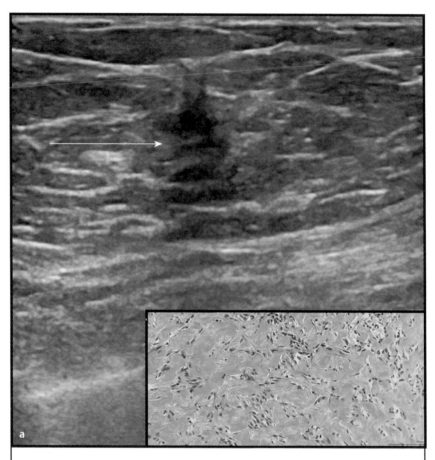

a

**Fig. 4.1 (a)** A 42-year old female with a palpable left breast mass. Ultrasound revealed an irregular hypoechoic lesion mimicking a breast carcinoma (*arrow*). Microphotograph shows pseudoangiomatous stromal hyperplasia with slit-like channels bordered by cells with no atypia (*inset*).

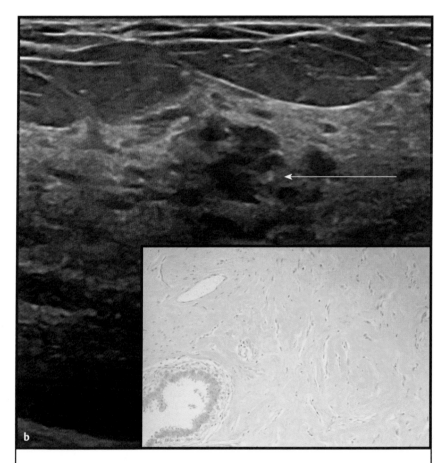

**Fig. 4.1 (b)** A 30-year-old female patient with diabetes type 1 and Grave's disease presented with a lump at 10 o'clock. Ultrasound revealed indeterminate, irregular, and hypoechoic lesion (*arrow*). Microphotograph showed anastomosing forming empty slit-vascular spaces (*inset*). There was no evidence of atypia. Abbreviation: PASH, pseudoangiomatous hyperplasia.

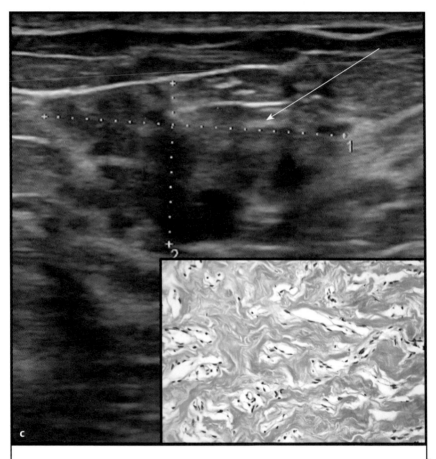

**Fig. 4.1 (c)** A 56-year-old female presented with a palpable lump within the central left breast. Ultrasound showed an irregular and hypoechoic 32 mm mass (*arrow*). This was suspicious for malignancy. Subsequent core biopsies and histopathological examination revealed pseudoangiomatous hyperplasia (*inset*).

# Sclerosing Adenosis

This is another interesting proliferative lesion which mainly involves terminal duct lobular unit. This benign condition can also present as malignant imaging characteristics and cause diagnostic dilemma. Sclerosing adenosis warrants thorough investigation as the appearances are nonspecific.

There is a wide range of clinical presentation like a small, tender, and firm nodule in the breast to often multiple nodules which become tender in the pre-perimenstrual period but majority of patients are asymptomatic.

Imaging features include an irregular mass on mammography (**Fig. 4.2a**), and ultrasound may demonstrate an irregular hypoechoic mass with or without distal acoustic shadowing (**Fig. 4.2b, d,** *arrows*).

Final diagnosis cannot be established on imaging in isolation and sinister pathology has to be excluded. This can be symptomatic and palpable; however, it is found accidentally in most cases on screening mammograms.

Smooth muscle actin immunohistochemistry highlights the presence of surrounding myoepithelial cells, confirming that the glands are benign (**Fig. 4.2c**).

Histology demonstrates proliferation of bilayered breast acini, some of which are compressed by a fibrotic stroma, obliterating the lumina of the glands. (**Fig. 4.2d,** *inset*)

The cause remains unknown. Even though this is a benign condition, some rare association with increased risk of developing breast cancer has been reported. This entity does not require any invasive treatment, however, may coexist with complex sclerosing lesions/ radial scars and excision may be encouraged.

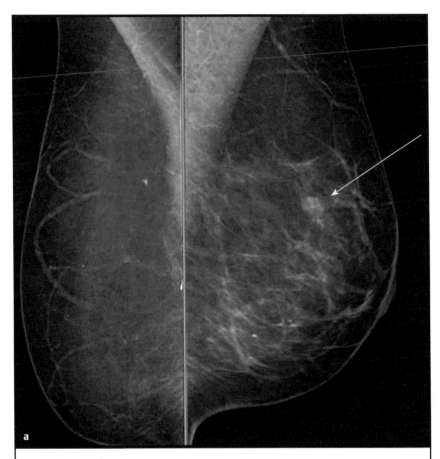

**Fig. 4.2 (a)** A 54-year old female who presented with a symptomatic lump within the upper left breast. Left MLO view shows an irregular mass (*arrow*). Abbreviation: MLO, mediolateral oblique.

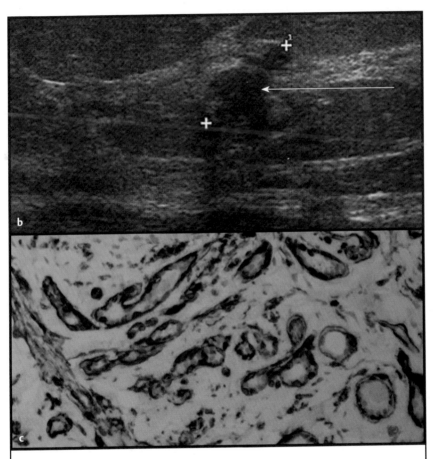

**Fig. 4.2 (b, c)** The same patient as in **Fig. 4.2a. (b)** Sonography showed a hypoechoic mass (*arrow*). This was irregular in shape and suspicious for malignancy. **(c)** Smooth muscle actin immunohistochemistry slide highlights the presence of surrounding myoepithelial cells, confirming that the glands are benign.

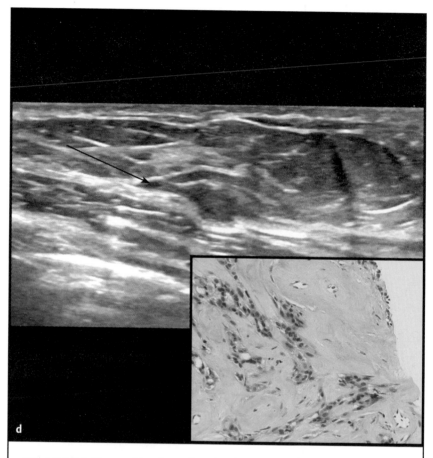

**Fig. 4.2 (d)** A 45-year-old patient referred to the triple breast assessment clinic with nodularity. Ultrasound scan showed incidental, subcentimeter, and hypoechoic lesion (*black arrow*). This was not palpable. Microphotograph showed features sclerosing adenosis with proliferation of bilayered breast acini, some of which are compressed by a fibrotic stroma, obliterating the lumina of the glands (*inset*).

# Complex Sclerosing Lesion/Radial Scar

This is a benign proliferative disorder and is often mistaken to be a sequel to postinflammation or postsurgical scarring, which is unrelated. Clinically nonpalpable, these lesions are usually picked up on screening mammograms.

Imaging can be a matter of concern for schirrhous carcinoma of breast. This can present as distortion and spiculate mass on mammography (**Fig. 4.3a**), with a low-density area in the core– classically described as the "Black star sign." Secondary changes like retraction with skin thickening are absent and act as a big hint toward diagnosis.

Sonography often reveals an irregular hypoechoic mass on ultrasound (**Fig. 4.3b**). Therefore, radiopathological correlation is the recommended line of investigation.

An example of radial scar on mammography shows close resemblance to malignancy (**Fig. 4.3c**). Breast radiologists often see such cases on screening; however, a complete workup can easily lead to the appropriate diagnosis.

The upgrade phenomenon is not high and management of complex sclerosing lesions still remains controversial.

Histology shows multiple ducts and lobules in radial configuration. The ducts and lobules can contain variable proliferative changes, for example, sclerosing adenosis or ductal hyperplasia (histologic image in **Fig. 4.3c**).

Central elastotic scar can be identified on histology.

This proliferative disorder is often labeled as "high-risk lesion" due to evidence of radial spicules/outgrowths on histology which is seen in many carcinomas.

Thus, excision is indicated to verify any potential atypical features or coexistence with malignancy or other high-risk lesions.

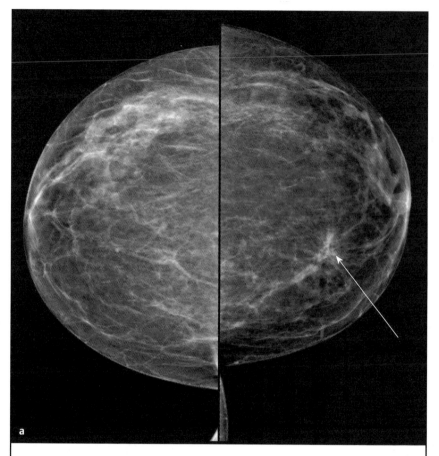

**Fig. 4.3 (a)** A 45-year-old female with a history of a symptomatic breast lump. Mammography and left CC view shows a spiculate mass with low density core (*arrow*). Abbreviation: CC, craniocaudal.

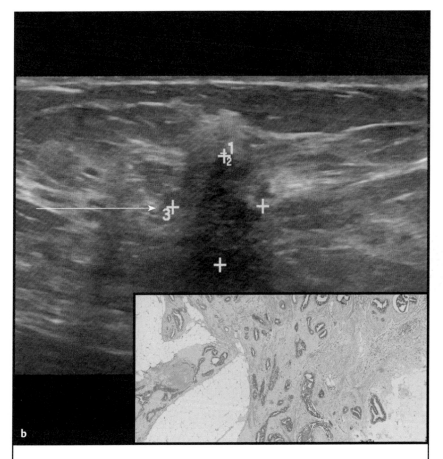

**Fig. 4.3 (b)** The same patient as in **Fig. 4.3a**. Ultrasound revealed an irregular and hypoechoic mass (*arrow*). This was taller than wide which added to the level of suspicion. Histology showed a complex sclerosing lesion (*inset*).

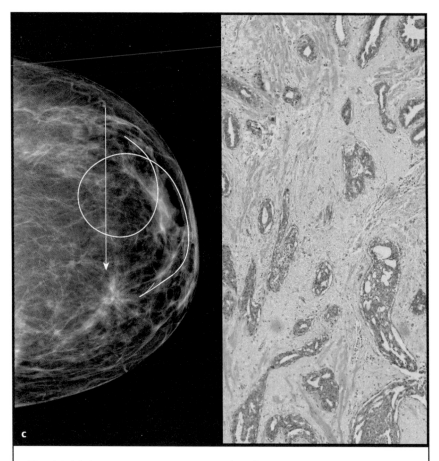

**Fig. 4.3 (c)** Same patient as in **Fig. 4.3a, b**. Left CC view shows wire localization of the histologically-proven complex sclerosing lesion (*long arrow*). Associated microphotograph (*right image*). Abbreviation: CC, craniocaudal.

# Epitheliosis of the Breast

This rare proliferative condition affects the breast ducts. This entity is also known as intraductal breast hyperplasia. Usual or conventional intraductal hyperplasia means that there is increased number of normal-appearing cells of mammary epithelium.

We illustrate an unusual example of epitheliosis in a young female patient who presented with a palpable breast lump. Ultrasound demonstrated irregular and hypoechoic mass (**Fig. 4.4a, b**). This was taller than its width, which significantly increased the level of suspicion. Imaging spectrum was highly suggestive of a carcinoma and the lesion was therefore assigned BI-RADS category 5.

Histopathology revealed epitheliosis of the breast with no evidence of atypia.

Various imaging characteristics have been associated with epitheliosis.

There are no pathognomonic—sonographic or mammographic—features that could guide us to the correct recognition, and microscopic examination is crucial to establish this diagnosis.

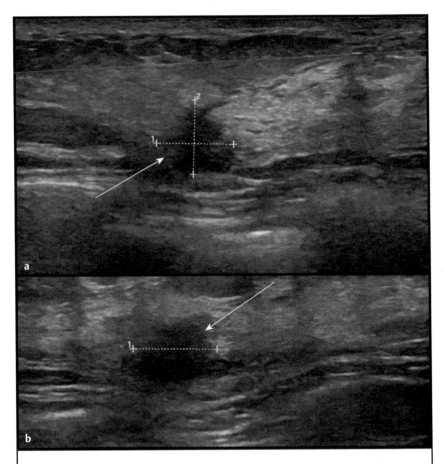

**Fig. 4.4 (a, b)** A 22-year-old female presented with some mild lumpiness within the central left breast. Ultrasound examination showed an irregular and hypoechoic mass (*arrows*) which raised suspicion of malignancy. Thus, multiple core biopsies were taken for verification.

**Points to Ponder**

*Proliferative conditions in breast are far more prevalent but are often mistaken for malignancy on imaging alone. For example, common benign counterparts like sclerosing adenosis, PASH, etc.*

*This reinstates the importance of image guided biopsies.*

# Bibliography

Adeniran A, Al-Ahmadie H, Mahoney MC, Robinson-Smith TM. Granular cell tumor of the breast: a series of 17 cases and review of the literature. Breast J 2004;10(6):528–531.

Chen Y-L, Chen J-J, Chang C, et al. Sclerosing adenosis: ultrasonographic and mammographic findings and correlation with histopathology. Mol Clin Oncol 2017;6(2): 157–162

Cohen MA, Newell MS. Radial scars of the breast encountered at core biopsy: review of histologic, imaging, and management considerations. AJR Am J Roentgenol 2017;209(5):1168–1177

Jaunoo SS, Thrush S, Dunn P. Pseudoangiomatous stromal hyperplasia (PASH): a brief review. Int J Surg 2011;9(1):20–22

Kennedy M, Masterson AV, Kerin M, Flanagan F. Pathology and clinical relevance of radial scars: a review. J Clin Pathol 2003;56(10):721–724

Kopans DB. Breast imaging. 3rd ed. Hagerstwon, MD: Lippincott Williams & Wilkins; 2007

Raju U, Crissman JD, Zarbo RJ, Gottlieb C. Epitheliosis of the breast. An immunohistochemical characterization and comparison to malignant intraductal proliferations of the breast. Am J Surg Pathol 1990;14(10):939–947

Shah BA, Mandawa SR. Breast Imaging A Core Review. 2nd ed. Philadelphia, PA: Wolters Kluwer; 2017

Tabar L, Dean PB. Teaching Atlas of Mammography. 4th ed. Thieme; 2011

Wegner U, Balschat S, Decker T, et al. Imaging findings of rare benign breast lesions: a pictorial review. Electronic Poster ECR; 2019

## Summary MCQs

### ■ Questions

Please choose true or false. More than one answer options may be correct.

*Question 1:* Which of the following statements regarding the presented cases are correct?

a)  Complex sclerosing lesion is a so-called "high-risk lesion."

b)  Pseudoangiomatous hyperplasia (PASH) is a malignant lesion.

c)  Pseudoangiomatous hyperplasia (PASH) is a so-called "high-risk lesion."

d)  Sclerosing adenosis has pathognomonic imaging features and does not require microscopic verification.

e)  Pseudoangiomatous hyperplasia (PASH) is a benign condition.

*Question 2:* Ultrasound and histology of sclerosing adenosis are shown. How would you describe sonographic findings?

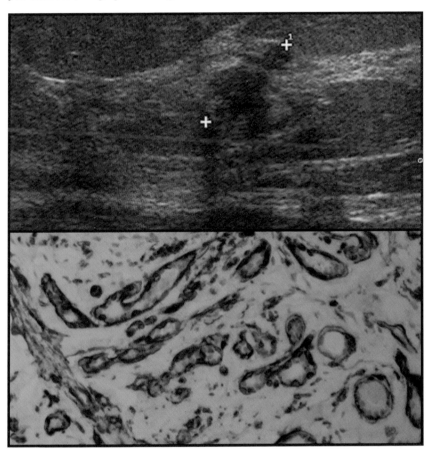

a)  Anechoic round lesion.

b)  Hyperechoic round subcutaneous lesion.

c)  A well-defined hypoechoic lesion.

d)  An irregular hypoechoic lesion.

e)  Normal.

**Question 3:** Ultrasound of the left breast is shown. Given, the presented sonographic features, what would be the next diagnostic step?

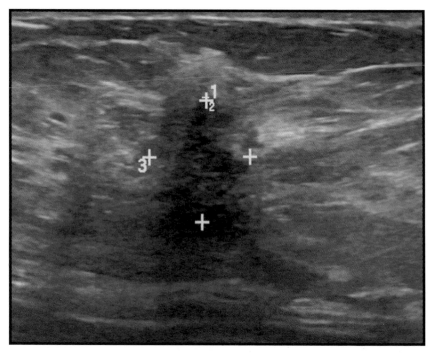

a)  No further management required.

b)  Ultrasound guided core needle biopsy.

c)  Breast magnetic resonance imaging (MRI).

d)  Stereotactic biopsy.

e)  Aspiration.

**Question 4:** Which of the following statements are correct?

a)  Lymphocytic mastopathy is associated with diabetes and autoimmune thyroid disease.

b)  Mammary sarcoidosis is a common manifestation of sarcoidosis.

c)  Tuberculous mastitis and idiopathic granulomatous mastitis are synonyms.

d)  Granular cell tumor (GCT) is a benign vascular tumor.

e)  Diabetic mastopathy may result in breast mass formation.

# ■ Answers

*Answer 1:*

a)  (T) Complex sclerosing lesion is a so-called "high-risk lesion" Thus, excision is encouraged to verify any potential atypical features or coexistence with malignancy or other high-risk lesions. The upgrade phenomenon is not high and management of complex sclerosing lesion still remains controversial.

b)  (F) Pseudoangiomatous hyperplasia (PASH) is a benign condition.

c)  (F) Pseudoangiomatous hyperplasia (PASH) is a benign lesion. This is not associated with increased risk or upgrade to malignancy.

d)  (F) Imaging findings of a sclerosing adenosis are nonspecific. This can mimic malignancy in breast radiology.

e)  (T) Pseudoangiomatous hyperplasia (PASH) is a benign stromal lesion in the setting of breast tissue overgrowth.

## References

Kopans DB. Breast imaging. 3rd ed. Hagerstwon, MD: Lippincott Williams & Wilkins; 2007

Shah BA, Mandawa SR. Breast Imaging A Core Review. 2nd ed. Philadelphia, PA: Wolters Kluwer; 2017

*Answer 2:*

a)  (F) This is neither anechoic nor round in shape.

b)  (F) Hyperechoic round subcutaneous lesion. Such description would be suggestive of a typical lipoma.

c)  (F) This is an irregular and hypoechoic lesion.

d)  (T) The sonographic mass is hypoechoic and irregular in shape.

e)  (F) An irregular hypoechoic mass is identified.

## Reference

Kopans DB. Breast imaging. 3rd ed. Hagerstwon, MD: Lippincott Williams & Wilkins; 2007

*Answer 3:*

a)  (F) Biopsy is required to exclude malignancy.

b)  (T) Ultrasound-guided core needle biopsy is the preferred next diagnostic step as microscopic verification is needed to establish the final diagnosis.

c)  (F) A solitary, solid mass on ultrasound is not an indication for MRI.

d)  (F) Stereotactic biopsy could be an option with regard to a mammographic abnormality.

e)  (F) This is a solid mass. No drainable collection identified.

## References

Kopans DB. Breast imaging. 3rd ed. Hagerstwon, MD: Lippincott Williams & Wilkins; 2007

Shah BA, Mandawa SR. Breast Imaging A Core Review. 2nd ed. Philadelphia, PA: Wolters Kluwer; 2017

*Answer 4:*

a)  (T) Lymphocytic mastopathy is associated with diabetes or various autoimmune diseases, for example, autoimmune thyroiditis.

b)  (F) Mammary sarcoidosis is not a common manifestation of sarcoidosis as it rarely occurs in the breast.

c)  (F) Tuberculous mastitis and idiopathic granulomatous mastitis are not synonyms; as tuberculous mastitis is a granulomatous disease caused by mycobacterium tuberculosis, whereas the cause of idiopathic granulomatous mastitis remains unknown.

d)  (F) Granular cell tumor (GCT) originates from Schwann cells.

e)  (T) Benign breast mass formation is a complication of long-standing diabetes.

## References

Kopans DB. Breast imaging. 3rd ed. Hagerstwon, MD: Lippincott Williams & Wilkins; 2007

Shah BA, Mandawa SR. Breast Imaging A Core Review. 2nd ed. Philadelphia, PA: Wolters Kluwer; 2017

# Miscellaneous Lesions

# Miscellaneous Lesions

## Learning Objectives:

1. To illustrate other potential conditions that could imitate malignant processes on either radiological or physical examination.

2. To broaden the perspective of breast radiologists with a few rare benign findings which resemble breast malignancies.

3. To summarize and empower new knowledge regarding the book, achieve success during the quiz, and obtain an excellent developmental feedback.

## Introduction

There are numerous other conditions which may result in a breast mass formation and give rise to misleading appearances on imaging or with regard to physical examination.

We will summarize some more common conditions such as fibroadenomas, hamartomas, fat necrosis, various complex collections within the breast, and sebaceous cysts.

We will also illustrate an unusual example of a benign salivary tumor within the breast as a curiosity.

# Fibroadenomas

These are very common and nonmalignant stromal breast lesions that mostly affect women in the second or third decade of life. Typical fibroadenomas have benign sonographic appearance and are usually round or oval in shape, homogenous, and hypoechoic with smooth margins.

Physical examination can reveal a palpable, smooth, and mobile mass.

Typical, simple fibroadenomas do not increase the risk of cancer and do not require surgical treatment. However, some fibroadenomas have atypical features on imaging which may cause diagnostic dilemma and uncertainty, namely, irregular margins, heterogeneous sonographic appearance, or large size manifesting as breast asymmetry or deformity. Sometimes the stromal calcifications within these fibroadenomas may be clustered on mammograms and require stereotactic biopsy for confirmation.

If the fibroadenomas are more than 5 cm or weigh more than 500 gm, they are labeled as juvenile giant fibroadenoma and can mimic phyllodes tumor (**Fig. 5.1a–d**).

Moreover, these lesions can contain coarse calcifications which produce posterior acoustic shadowing that can mimic malignancy on ultrasound.

Atypical fibroadenomas may be larger in size, sonographically heterogenous and contain multiple cystic spaces (**Fig. 5.1e–g**).

Furthermore, these solid masses can either be solitary or multicentric. With regard to atypical cases, carcinoma of the breast or phyllodes tumor are one of the main differentials and can be identified via ultrasound-guided biopsy.

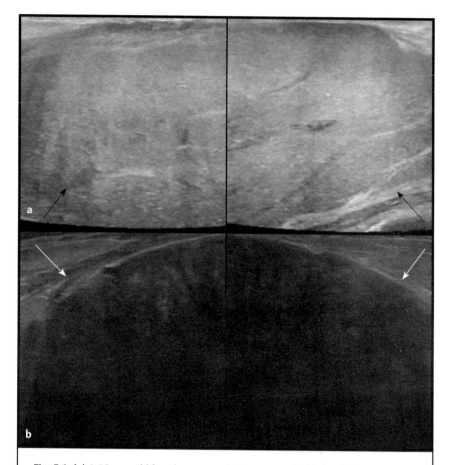

**Fig. 5.1 (a)** A 16-year old female presented with a new palpably hard left breast mass (*black arrows*). This was suspicious on physical examination. Ultrasound revealed a solitary, well-defined mass involving most of the affected breast. This mass was difficult to fully measure in a single window concerning a phyllodes tumor as a main differential. Subsequent excisional biopsy revealed an entirely benign, giant, juvenile fibroadenoma. **(b)** The image demonstrates a similar case of a giant juvenile fibroadenoma in a different symptomatic 10-year old patient female (*white arrows*). The mass involved the whole right breast and was difficult to measure. This was fully excised and total weight was approximately 1000 g.

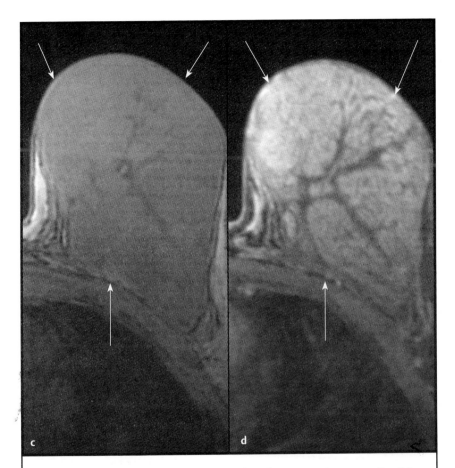

**Fig. 5.1 (c, d)** MRI of the breast with regard to the same patient as on **Fig. 5.1a.**
**(c)** T1-weighted sequence without fat saturation shows a large, smoothly marginated
hypointense mass. This involves almost the entire left breast, causing asymmetry and
deformity. **(d)** T1-weighted postcontrast sequence shows bright enhancement of the
mass. This contains clearly evident nonenhancing septations which is a quite common
feature regarding fibroadenomas. Abbreviation: MRI, magnetic resonance imaging.

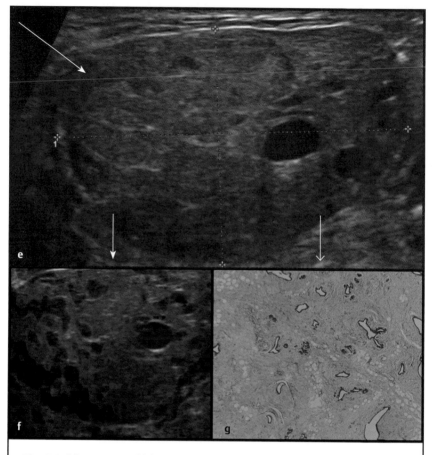

**Fig. 5.1 (e)** A 15-year old female presented with a new palpably hard right breast mass (*long arrow*). Ultrasound revealed a solitary, well-defined mass involving the 12 o' clock position of right breast. This mass had smooth margins but multiple cystic spaces could be seen within it. **(f)** Elastography showed moderately soft consistency with a normal footprint (*short arrow*). **(g)** Subsequent excisional biopsy revealed an atypical fibroadenoma with plenty of fibroblasts and slit-like spaces as seen in the microphotograph (*arrowhead*).

# Fat Necrosis

This benign process represents injured breast tissue in the setting of posttraumatic changes, a sequela of surgery, or other invasive procedures. This may be a challenge due to its variable imaging spectrum. Clinically, fat necrosis can present as a palpable lump, skin thickening with or without associated bruising, or even rarely retraction in subacute stages.

Imaging findings may cause uncertainty, especially in the patients who do not report any history of trauma. Fat necrosis demonstrates no flow on Doppler. On imaging, fat necrosis can result in solid-appearing mass formation, cystic degeneration, or even complex solid–cystic masses (**Fig. 5.2a, b**). Subtle avascular wall nodularity toward the inner aspect of the cystic component needs careful observation and can lead to diagnosis.

Doppler application can help us distinguish this condition from carcinoma as the latter may show Doppler flow with regard to solid-appearing components (**Fig. 5.2c, d**).

In fact, this benign condition can mimic both intracystic malignancy or complex inflammatory change (**Fig. 5.2e–g**).

Mammography usually reveals oil cysts and these may also contain focal dense nodules or thick walls (**Fig. 5.2h**). Subacute cases may also show flecks of calcifications apart from soap bubble-like calcifications, appearing similar to ductal carcinoma in situ (DCIS).

It is important to know that calcifications within the fat necrosis change over time and can be compared easily on serial mammograms.

Histology of core biopsy samples clearly reveals liquefactive fat necrosis with few areas of hemorrhage in acute phase, followed by fibroblasts and scarring as sequelae.

Fat necrosis is the result of liquified fatty tissue and subsequent fibrosis, does not require surgical interventions, and the overall prognosis is excellent.

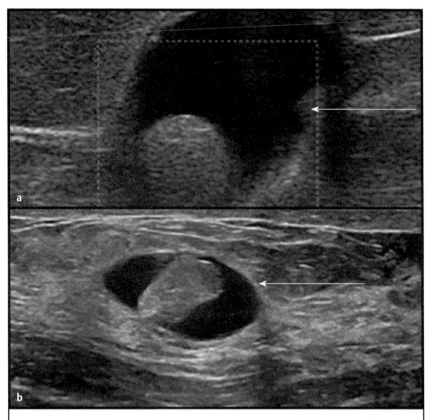

**Fig. 5.2 (a, b)** Ultrasound demonstrates examples of fat necrosis (*white arrows*) There are homogenously hyperechoic avascular components within the cystic area in the breast.

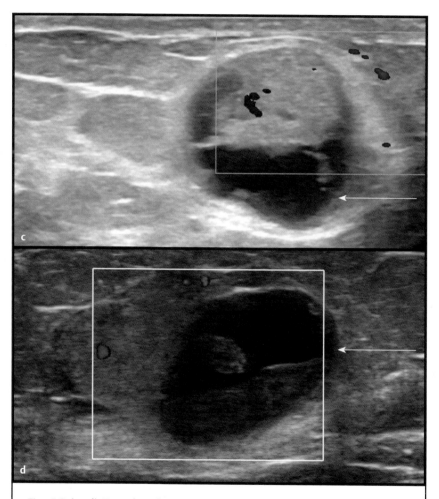

**Fig. 5.2 (c, d)** Examples of mucinous carcinoma (*arrows*). Solid components of cancerous lesions are irregular in shape and can show flow on Doppler application as opposed to avascular and more smoothly marginated fat necrosis.

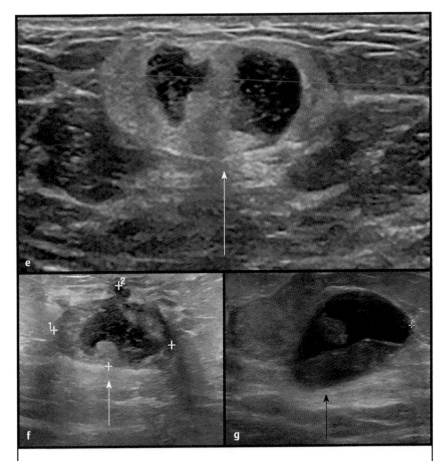

**Fig. 5.2 (e–g)** Diagnostic challenges on sonography. Comparison slide shows two an example of fat necrosis (*white arrow* in **e**) versus idiopathic granulomatous mastitis (*white arrow* in **f**) versus mucinous carcinoma (*black arrow* in **g**). Please note that all entities may have shared imaging features and contain both solid-appearing and fluid-like components.

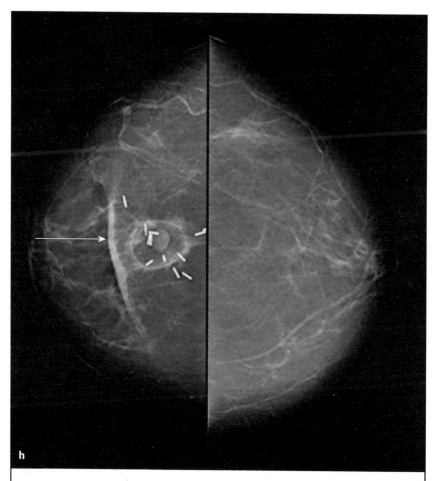

h

**Fig. 5.2 (h)** Bilateral mammogram, craniocaudal view. Surveillance following wide local excision of malignancy. This is an example of one of the most typical appearances of fat necrosis on mammography. Oil cyst with a dense rim and a centrally located rounded nodule (*arrow*).

# Hamartomas

Hamartomas are entirely benign breast masses which can form in the setting of breast tissue overgrowth. Interestingly, the term "hamartomas" was first used for these breast lesions by Arrigoni et al in 1971 (previously known as fibrolipomas). Fibroadenolipoma or "breast within the breast" lesions are other medical descriptors, and these can be used synonymously. The age group of involvement in hamartomas is usually above 35 years, and patients also present with painless lump which coincides with most cancers and creates a confusing picture.

Mammography shows rounded, well-circumscribed opacity with a thin rim of pseudocapsule. There is an interplay of radiolucent and radiodense components within the mass, representing fatty and stromal components (**Fig. 5.3d**).

Localizing hamartomas on ultrasound is often difficult and needs trained eyes to demarcate the margins as they merge really well with the rest of the breast parenchyma (**Fig. 5.3c**) They can have ill-defined margins and irregular, hypoechoic as well as hyperechoic contents on gray-scale ultrasound (**Fig. 5.3b**)

These lesions can be palpable and sometimes demonstrate variable misleading appearances closely resembling a poorly-defined mass (**Fig. 5.3e** and **Fig. 5.3a**, *arrows*)

Postcore biopsy and microscopic verification can exclude malignancy in cases of uncertainty.

Histopathology demonstrates unremarkable breast tissue in keeping with benign etiology. No surgical interventions are required.

Routine follow-up depending on further symptoms may be considered as carcinoma may arise in hamartomas as in any other breast tissue.

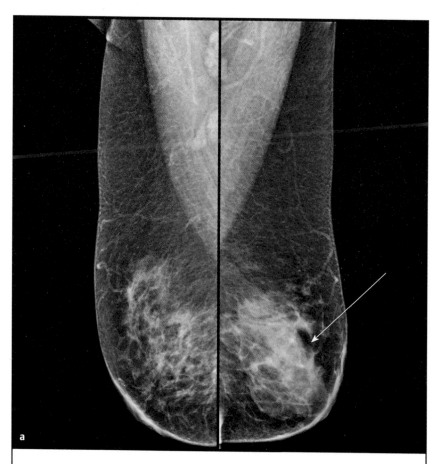

**Fig. 5.3 (a)** Bilateral mammography. MLO view shows a heterogeneous mass with some radiolucent components (*arrow*). This is partially ill-defined without any overt pseudocapsule. This was palpable and subsequent multiple ultrasound-guided core biopsies confirmed hamartoma. Abbreviation: MLO, mediolateral oblique.

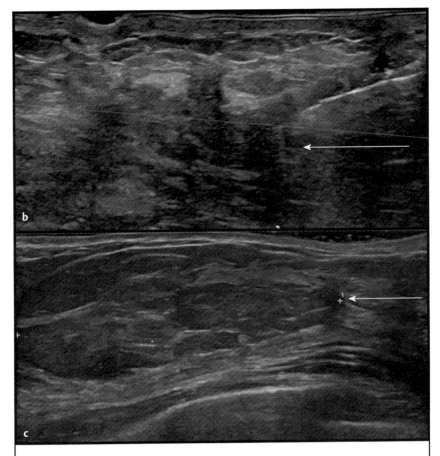

**Fig. 5.3 (b, c)** Comparison slide demonstrates atypical and typical sonographic appearances of a hamartoma. Typical hamartoma/fibroadenolipoma (*arrow* in **c**) resembles normal breast tissue and contains both fibroglandular and fatty components. Moreover, this was palpable and ovoid in shape. A subtle pseudocapsule can be seen (also, see the associated mammographic correlate with pathognomonic appearance on **Fig. 5.3d**). The other atypical-appearing and biopsy-proven hamartoma (*arrow* in **b**) demonstrated ill-defined margins and consisted of irregular, hypoechoic as well as hyperechoic contents. No overt pseudocapsule was visualized on ultrasound. Moreover, this was palpable on examination. Thus, ultrasound is not always helpful in establishing the diagnosis. Please see associated mammographic correlate on **Fig. 5.3e**.

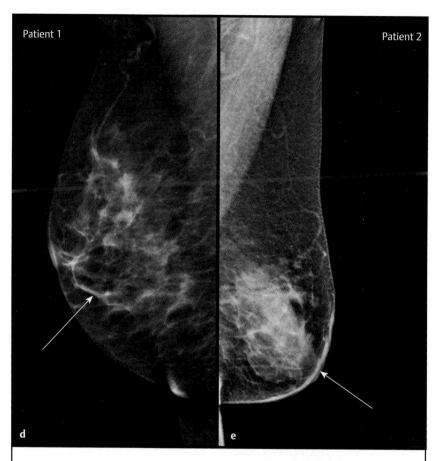

Patient 1

Patient 2

d

e

**Fig. 5.3 (d, e)** Two different patients are shown. Comparison slide demonstrates typical hamartoma (**d**) and atypical hamartoma (**e**). The latter mimics a suspicious mass on mammography. Typical hamartoma (*arrow* in **d**) correlates with the same patient as on **Fig. 5.3c**. This reveals an ovoid heterogenous lesion with a pseudocapsule and prominent, radiolucent fatty components. Atypical hamartoma (*arrow* in **e**) correlates with the same patient as on **Fig. 5.3b**. This also contains radiolucent, more fatty components. However, this lesion is much denser and partially ill-defined.

## Complex Benign Masses such as Chronic Seromas, Hematomas, Abscesses, Other Inflammatory Collections or Complicated Cysts

Chronic seromas may cause confusion on various imaging modalities and can manifest as cystic, with thick irregular septations in mature collections. Potentially, more solid-appearing components can be seen within the collections, indicating debris. Color Doppler shows absent flow within debris and helps in differentiating it from nodular soft-tissue component in malignancies.

For example, invasive carcinoma can demonstrate appearances similar to benign postoperative seromas (**Fig. 5.4a–c**). In addition, breast abscess may mimic inflammatory carcinoma and present as palpable irregular masses (**Fig. 5.4d–f**).

Hematomas as a result of local trauma, biopsy or even secondary to coagulopathy, or seat belt injury can easily appear like malignancy and confuse even a well-practiced radiologist if proper referral or history is not provided. Mammography may show mass or simply an area of increased parenchymal density—the second type is often diagnostically challenging.

Serial ultrasounds make diagnosis easier as the hematoma starts showing changes consistent with fat necrosis and then starts to gradually organize and scar.

Breast abscesses are commonly seen in lactating women as a complication of mastitis. One should be also aware that nonpuerperal breast abscesses in chronic smokers or diabetic patients can resemble carcinoma.

As ultrasound is the primary modality for confirmation, few salient points can be considered while doing the scan. An abscess will show a multiloculated collection with distal acoustic enhancement due to fluid within the abscess cavity (**Fig. 5.4e, f**).

The peripheral rim of vascular congestion may also resemble neovascularization in malignancies but will lack the low-resistance pattern on spectral Doppler, which is seen in association with neovascularization of malignancies due to absence of elastic tissue in these vessels.

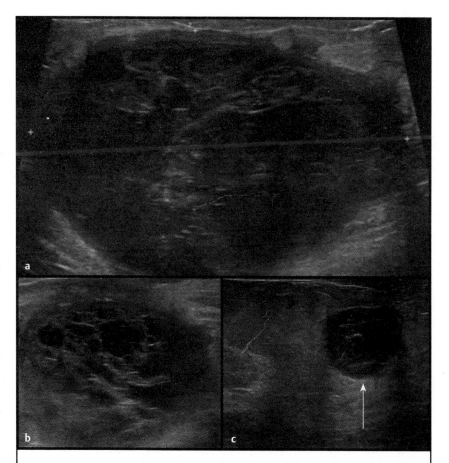

**Fig. 5.4 (a–c)** Comparison slide and challenges of ultrasound examination. Examples of benign chronic collections and seromas following surgery **(a, b)**. Invasive ductal carcinoma of no special type grade 2 (*arrow* in **c**). Please note that both malignancy and its mimics have shared imaging features in keeping with solid-appearing and fluid-like components.

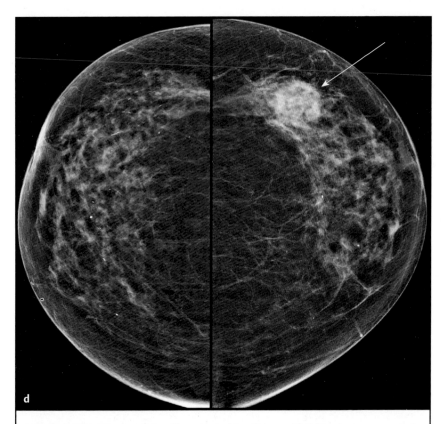

**Fig. 5.4 (d)** A 76-year old female patient with a history of left hip abscess presented with a new palpably hard and clinically suspicious breast mass. Mammography showed irregular lesion within the left outer breast (*arrow*).

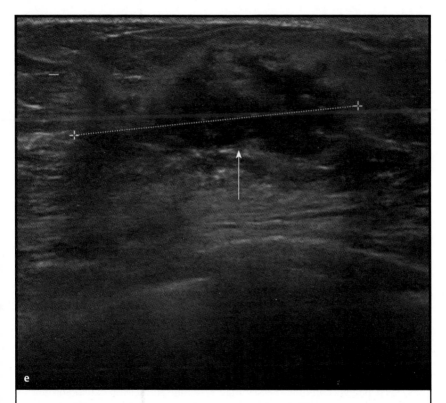

e

**Fig. 5.4 (e)** Breast abscess or malignancy– a potential dilemma on sonography. The image represents the same patient as in **Fig. 5.4d**. Subsequent ultrasound demonstrated irregular hypoechoic mass (*arrow*). This was highly suspicious for malignancy, thus assigned BI-RADS 5. The ipsilateral axilla was normal. Multiple core biopsies were performed and the lesion collapsed during sampling. Histology revealed an abscess which is one of the common malignancy mimics. Abbreviation: BI-RADS, breast imaging reporting and database system score.

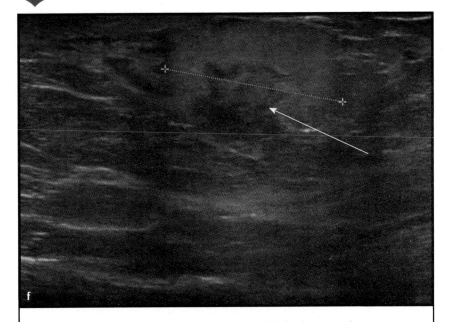

**Fig. 5.4 (f)** A 39-year-old female with a new, palpably hard mass in the upper outer quadrant of the left breast. Ultrasound revealed an irregular predominantly hypoechoic mass (*arrow*). This was mistaken for a carcinoma both on initial physical examination and ultrasound scan. However, core biopsies and subsequent histology demonstrated an abscess. Moreover, the lesion collapsed during sampling and the patient had a history of infected nipple piercing.

Thus, such benign complex masses may resemble intracystic carcinoma during gray-scale ultrasound examination and may warrant microscopic verification.

In such situations, a detailed history and progression of disease can help the radiologist while doing the scans. Doppler and ultrasound elastography is used to evaluate the vascularity and disease footprint for drawing conclusions.

However, surgical excision of complex solid–cystic masses may sometimes be considered in cases concerning medical history or technically difficult sampling.

Clinical scenario can help us avoid unnecessary interventions, for example, a residual hematoma with echogenic debris or septations, following recent surgery, can be easily followed-up and no biopsies are necessary.

Please note that with regard to the presented patients, it is not possible to exclude a carcinoma, based on imaging alone.

## Mimics for Metastatic Lymphadenopathy

This topic can be again commonly encountered by breast radiologists, but in this chapter, we shall emphasize on the less discussed mimics of lymphadenopathy which are rare but need consideration in the complicated scenarios.

Tattoo pigment particles can easily migrate into the lymphatic system with regard to the drainage areas in the acute phase, but very few case reports have proven similar reaction in chronic phase also.

This subsequently causes inflammation with cortical thickening and enlargement of regional lymph nodes (**Fig. 5.5a**, *arrow*). Histology shows pigment-laden macrophages; red pigment in our case as the lady had a red dragon for tattoo (**Fig. 5.5a**, *inset*).

Although pathologists recommend further evaluation by immunohistochemistry, certain radiological features should definitely be mentioned while reporting, including the shape of lymph node and the architecture despite the enlargement and cortical thickening.

Benign conditions such as sarcoid or reactionary lymph nodes secondary to infections, allergies, or foreign substance reactions can easily imitate metastatic spread to the lymphatic system or simulate breast-related malignancy (**Fig. 5.5b–d**).

The heavy metal component of the tattoo ink can be deposited into the lymph node sinus or phagocytosed by the macrophages. This may appear as pleomorphic calcifications in the axillary region on mammograms which are often biopsied.

Apart from common infective causes, it is important to highlight the phenomenon of secondary reactionary lymph nodes; in particular, the setting of the increasing trend of tattooing.

Since decorative emblems of the skin have become more popular, the associated adverse reactions can also more frequently cause potential medical dilemmas.

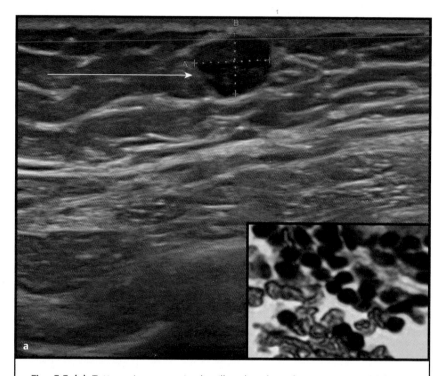

**Fig. 5.5 (a)** Tattoo pigment stained axillary lymph nodes. A 28-year old female presented with palpable lumpiness within the left axilla. Ultrasound showed well-defined hypoechoic lesions, mimicking abnormal lymph nodes and concerning for malignancy (*arrow*). Subsequent core biopsies and histology revealed reactionary lymph node with multiple red tattoo pigment deposits (*inset*). Patient had a red dragon tattoo at the level of ipsilateral scapula, and the colorful ink has leaked into the lymphatic system, appearing within macrophages in axillary node cores.

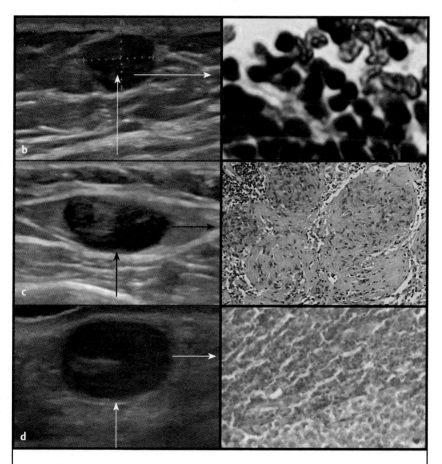

**Fig. 5.5 (b–d)** (top to bottom with corresponding histology): Interesting comparison regarding tattoo pigment-induced reactionary lymphadenopathy (*long white arrows* in **b**) versus mammary sarcoidosis (*short black arrows* in **c**) versus metastatic breast cancer lymph nodes (*short white arrows* in **d**). Metastatic lymphadenopathy and its benign mimics share very similar spectrum of imaging features as illustrated above. Resultant reactionary lymphadenopathy (**c**) can be indistinguishable from metastatic breast cancer nodal disease (*short white arrows* in **d**).

# Pleomorphic Adenoma of the Breast

It is an indolent salivary tumor. This is also known as a benign mixed tumor.

Location in the breast is very rare, as this most commonly occurs in a parotid gland.

This usually presents as a slowly growing, solitary mass which is indistinguishable from a carcinoma and can affect both sexes.

Ultrasound may show an irregular and hypoechoic mass (**Fig. 5.6a**, *arrow*). The location is deeper to the skin and is not superficial.

Mammography may show an irregular and relatively dense opacity (**Fig. 5.6c**)

These tumors can be easily diagnosed via ultrasound-guided core biopsy.

Histologically, this can have variable, pleomorphic appearance.

Histology of the cores shows dense myxomatous stroma with embedded myoepithelial and epithelial cells (**Fig. 5.6b**).

Benign mixed tumor of the breast can recur and also carries minimal risk of malignant transformation.

Therefore, wide local excision with clear margins, in order to avoid recurrence, is warranted.

Since it is one of the least common tumors of the breast, it may cause a real diagnostic challenge and mislead dedicated breast imagers. The exact etiology remains unknown.

The prognosis with regard to rare benign mixed tumor of the breast is very good.

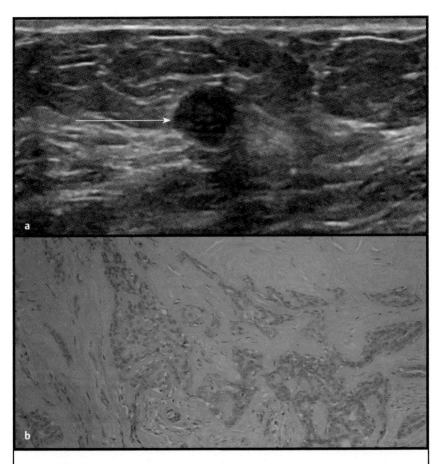

**Fig. 5.6 (a)** Ultrasound revealed an irregular and hypoechoic mass, concerning for a carcinoma (*arrow*). Therefore, this was assigned BI-RADS 5. **(b)** Microphotograph showed features of a benign salivary tumor in keeping with a pleomorphic adenoma. Pathology revealed a lesion with a central zone of chondroid differentiation. At the edges of the cartilage, there are proliferations of ductal-type epithelium with bilayered ducts. Abbreviation: BI-RADS, breast imaging reporting and database system score.

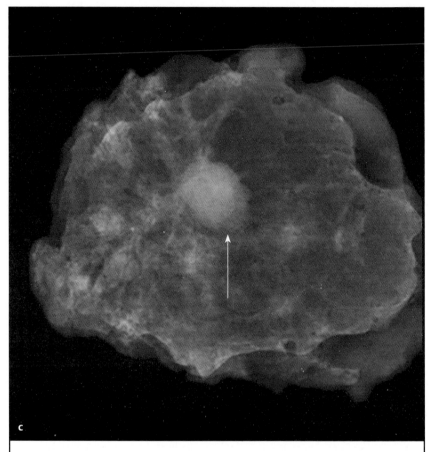

**Fig. 5.6 (c)** This is the same patient as on **Fig. 5.6a, b**. Wide local excision specimen of excised pleomorphic adenoma (*arrow*).

# Breast Sebaceous Cysts or Epidermal Inclusion Cysts

These very rarely cause any diagnostic dilemma, as they usually have typical imaging features and are located within subcutaneous tissues.

Ultrasound examination commonly reveals a superficially located, hypoechoic mass (**Fig. 5.7a, b;** *arrows*).

In some cases, a small sinus track extending toward the skin can be visualized (**Fig. 5.7a,** *short arrow*).

In contrast, the illustrated pleomorphic adenoma of the breast does not have a sinus tract and its location is not subcutaneous (**Fig. 5.7c,** *white arrow* in top right image). This benign tumor was irregular in shape and indistinguishable from a carcinoma on imaging; therefore, assigned breast imaging reporting and database system (BI-RADS) 5.

Please note associated microphotographs (**Fig. 5.7b, c;** bottom images).

However, sebaceous cysts of the breast can present as palpably hard lumps, cause anxiety in symptomatic patients, and also sometimes cause confusion on imaging.

While the shape can be variable and misleading, the pathognomonic sinus track and location beneath the skin are very helpful in establishing the diagnosis.

Sebaceous cyst may become inflamed and painful and require removal. These are totally benign, there is no association with increased risk of breast cancer, and the subsequent prognosis is excellent.

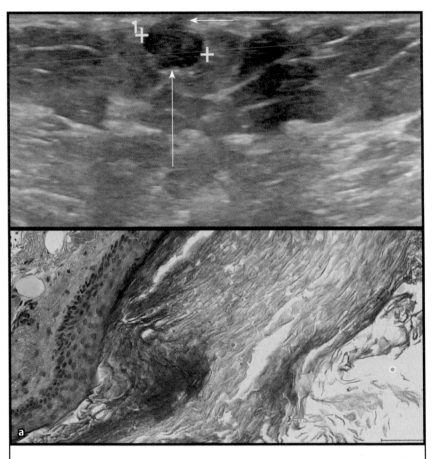

**Fig. 5.7 (a)** A symptomatic 36-year old female patient presented to the breast unit with a new palpable lump within the upper outer quadrant of the left breast. Sonography showed a hypoechoic subcutaneous mass (*top image, long arrow*). Please note subtle sinus tract extending towards the skin surface (*short arrow*). Histology confirmed a benign sebaceous cyst (*bottom image*). There was no evidence of malignancy.

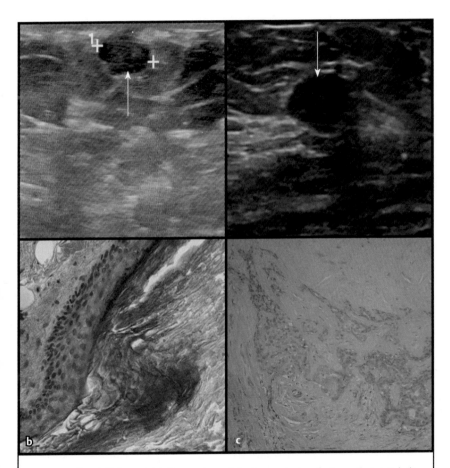

**Fig. 5.7 (b, c)** (*left to right*) Comparison slide demonstrates features that can help you diagnose a sebaceous cyst and distinguish it from other entities. Ultrasound examination shows a hypoechoic sebaceous cyst **(b)**. This is located beneath the skin and also has a sinus tract which extends toward the skin (*white arrow*). Sinus tract and location can help to differentiate this entity from a carcinoma Please note that pleomorphic adenoma **(c)** is located deeper and no sinus tract is observed..

## Points to Ponder

*Abscess, chronic hematoma, seroma, or malignancy can share similar imaging features and contain both fluid-like and more solid-appearing components.*

*Even equipped with a broad knowledge of variables and benign entities in breast imaging, it is often not possible to establish the diagnoses based on imaging alone.*

*Histopathological verification usually represents a gold standard of the diagnostic pathway, as it can help us to verify radiology and exclude a malignant process.*

# Bibliography

Arrigoni MG, Dockerty MB, Judd ES. The identification and treatment of mammary hamartomas. Surg Gynecol Obstet 1971;133:577–582

Doshi DJ, March DE, Crisi GM, Coughlin BF. Complex cystic breast masses: diagnostic approach and imaging-pathologic correlation. Radiographics 2007;27(Suppl 1): S53–S64

Ginter PS, Scognamiglio T, Tauchi-Nishi P, Antonio LB, Hoda SA. Pleomorphic adenoma of breast: a radiological and pathological study of a common tumor in an uncommon location. Case Rep Pathol 2015;2015:172750

Jack CM, Adwani A, Krishnan H. Tattoo pigment in an axillary lymph node simulating metastatic malignant melanoma. Int Semin Surg Oncol 2005;2:28

Kopans DB. Breast imaging. 3rd ed. Hagerstwon, MD: Lippincott Williams & Wilkins; 2007

Pluguez-Turull CW, Nanyes JE, Quintero CJ, et al. Idiopathic granulomatous mastitis: manifestations at multimodality imaging and pitfalls. Radiographics 2018;38: 330–356

Shah BA, Mandawa SR. Breast Imaging A Core Review. 2nd ed. Philadelphia, PA: Wolters Kluwer; 2017

Spratt JD, Salkowski LR, Loukas M, et al. Weir & Abrahams' Imaging Atlas of Human Anatomy. 5th ed. Elsevier; 2016

Tabar L, Dean PB. Teaching Atlas of Mammography. 4th ed. Thieme; 2011

## Summary MCQs

### ■ Questions

Please choose true or false. More than one answer option may be correct.

*Question 1:* Which of the following statements are correct?

a) Giant fibroadenoma is a common variant of a fibroadenoma in elderly patients.

b) Hamartoma and fibroadenolipoma represent the same entity and both medical descriptors can be used synonymously.

c) Fat necrosis of the breast requires surgical treatment due to its malignant potential.

d) Pleomorphic adenoma of the breast is a common breast tumor.

e) Fatty components of breast hamartomas may appear as radiolucent areas on mammography.

*Question 2:* Pleomorphic adenoma of the left breast is shown. How would you describe sonographic findings?

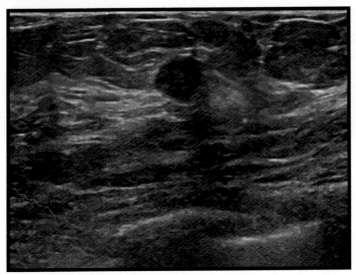

a) Anechoic round lesion.

b) Hyperechoic, round subcutaneous lesion.

c) A well-defined hypoechoic lesion.

d) An irregular hypoechoic lesion.

e) Normal.

*Question 3:* Which shape indicates mammographic abnormality?

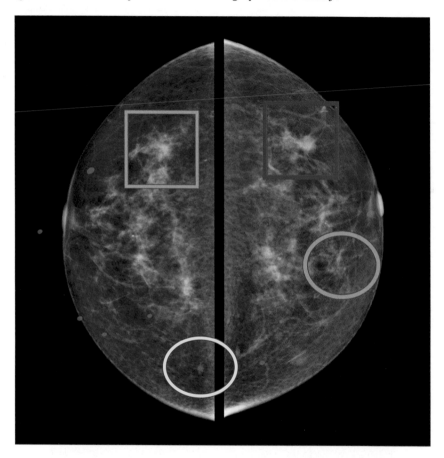

a) Blue square.

b) Red square.

c) Yellow circle.

d) Green circle.

*Question 4:* Fat necrosis and intracystic carcinoma are shown. Which figures are more likely to represent fat necrosis and which ones could rather represent malignancy?

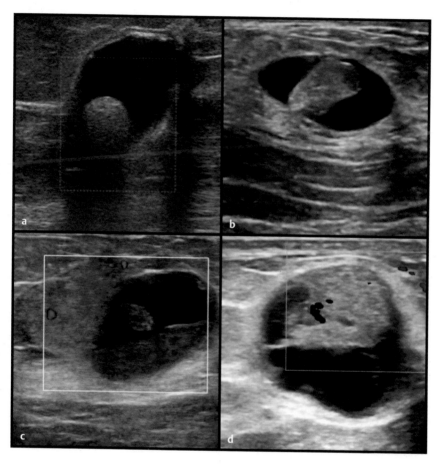

a) **Figs. c** and **d** are more likely to represent fat necrosis.

b) **Figs. a** and **c** are more likely represent fat necrosis.

c) All figures most likely demonstrate fat necrosis.

d) **Figs. a** and **b** are more likely to represent fat necrosis.

e) **Figs. b** and **d** are more likely to represent fat necrosis.

**Question 5:** What are the sonographic features that could potentially help you distinguish malignancy from fat necrosis?

a) Fat necrosis can demonstrate flow on Doppler application.

b) Breast cancer can demonstrate flow on Doppler application.

c) Breast carcinoma usually has more irregular margins.

d) Fat necrosis usually has more irregular margins.

e) None of the above.

**Question 6:** Epitheliosis of the left breast is shown. Please match the *arrows* with correct anatomical structures.

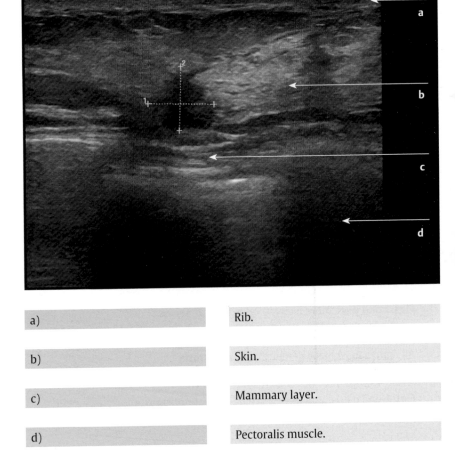

a)                                              Rib.

b)                                              Skin.

c)                                              Mammary layer.

d)                                              Pectoralis muscle.

**Question 7:** Which of the following statements are correct?

a) Fat necrosis is commonly associated with a history of trauma.

b) Intracystic malignancy of the breast and fat necrosis can have shared imaging features.

c) Diabetic mastopathy and lymphocytic mastopathy have different spectrum of histopathological features.

d) Mammary sarcoidosis is a common manifestation with regard to systemic sarcoidosis.

e) Free silicone can induce foreign body granulomatous mastitis.

**Question 8:** Bilateral and biopsy-proven diabetic mastopathy is shown. Given the final benign diagnosis, what is the appropriate BI-RADS assessment?

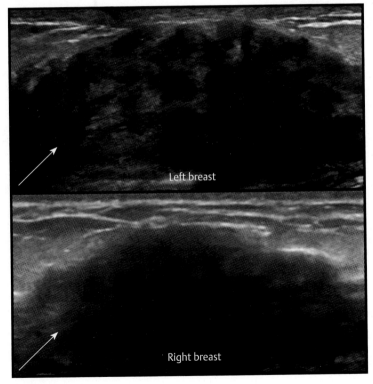

a) BI-RADS 5.

b) BI-RADS 1.

c) BI-RADS 2.

d) BI-RADS 4.

**Question 9:** Granular cell tumor of the breast is shown. How would you describe the associated mammographic abnormality?

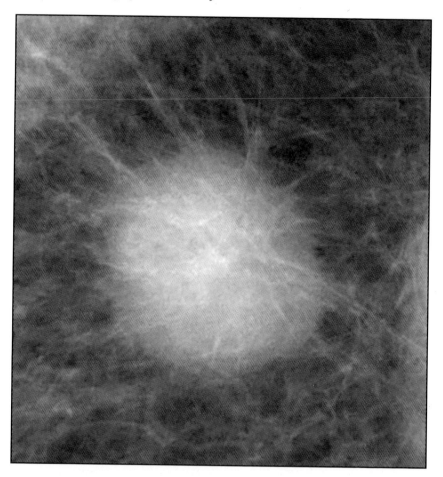

a) Oval lesion with extensive halo sign.

b) Architectural distortion.

c) No significant findings identified.

d) Microcalcifications.

e) High density lesion with spicules.

*Question 10:* Ultrasound examination of the left breast is demonstrated. What would be your next diagnostic step?

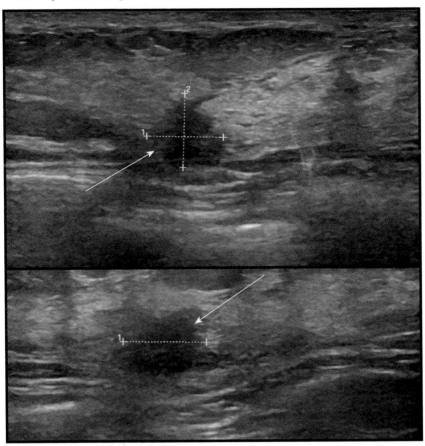

a) No further management required.

b) Ultrasound guided core needle biopsy.

c) Breast magnetic resonance imaging (MRI).

d) Stereotactic biopsy.

e) Aspiration.

# ■ Answers

*Answer 1:*

a)  (F) Giant fibroadenoma is a rare variant of a fibroadenoma and usually develops in younger women.

b)  (T) Mammary hamartoma is also known as fibroadenolipoma. This can also be described as "breast within the breast" lesion.

c)  (F) Fat necrosis within the breast is an entirely benign condition associated with trauma or surgery.

d)  (F) Pleomorphic adenoma is one of the least common breast neoplasms. This most commonly occurs in salivary glands.

e)  (T) Mammary hamartomas contain both fatty and fibroglandular breast tissue. Fatty tissue is radiolucent on mammography. Some hamartomas may have atypical appearance due to decreased amount of fat and subsequently resemble a more solid mass. Moreover, the associated pseudocapsule is not well visualized in some cases.

## References

Ginter PS, Scognamiglio T, Tauchi-Nishi P, Antonio LB, Hoda SA. Pleomorphic adenoma of breast: a radiological and pathological study of a common tumor in an uncommon location. Case Rep Pathol 2015;2015:172750

Kopans DB. Breast imaging. 3rd ed. Hagerstwon, MD: Lippincott Williams & Wilkins; 2007

*Answer 2:*

a)  (F) The lesion is neither anechoic nor round in shape.

b)  (F) Hyperechoic, round subcutaneous lesion are the features of a typical lipoma.

c)  (F) This is an irregular and hypoechoic lesion.

d)  (T) The sonographic mass is hypoechoic and irregular in shape.

e)  (F) An irregular hypoechoic mass is identified.

## Reference

Kopans DB. Breast imaging. 3rd ed. Hagerstwon, MD: Lippincott Williams & Wilkins; 2007

*Answer 3:*

a)   (F) Blue square represents parenchymal asymmetry but lacks distortion and has smooth margins with density similar to remaining parenchyma. This likely represents a glandular island.

b)   (T) Red square represents pathological area as there is parenchymal distortion along with asymmetry. Also, the density is relatively increased due to nodule formation.

c)   (F) Yellow circle represents a tiny, smooth margin opacity and has low-density likely to represent a benign pathology like a skin lesion (tag or a mole).

d)   (F) Green circle represents benign breast tissue.

## References

Doshi DJ, March DE, Crisi GM, Coughlin BF. Complex cystic breast masses: diagnostic approach and imaging-pathologic correlation. Radiographics 2007;27(Suppl 1): S53–S64

Kopans DB. Breast imaging. 3rd ed. Hagerstwon, MD: Lippincott Williams & Wilkins; 2007

*Answer 4:*

a)   (F) No, **Figs. c** and **d** are unlikely to represent fat necrosis due to Doppler flow with regard to solid-appearing components. These are highly suspicious for malignancy.

b)   (F) No, **Fig. c** unlikely represents fat necrosis due to Doppler flow with regard to solid-appearing component.

c)   (F) Not all figures demonstrate fat necrosis. **Figs. c** and **d** are most likely intracystic carcinomas due to Doppler flow with regard to solid-appearing components.

d)   (T) **Figs. a** and **b** are more likely to represent fat necrosis. These are smoothly marginated lesions with both solid-appearing and fluid-like components. In addition, there is no flow on Doppler application.

e)   (F) **Fig. d** does not represent fat necrosis as there is flow with regard to its solid-appearing components.

# References

Doshi DJ, March DE, Crisi GM, Coughlin BF. Complex cystic breast masses: diagnostic approach and imaging-pathologic correlation. Radiographics 2007;27(Suppl 1): S53–S64

Kopans DB. Breast Imaging. 3rd ed

*Answer 5:*

a) (F) Fat necrosis has no flow on Doppler application.

b) (T) Breast cancer can demonstrate flow on Doppler application due to neoangiogenesis.

c) (T) Breast carcinoma usually has more irregular margins due to microlobulation and irregular growth in tumor cells along with absence of capsulation.

d) (F) Fat necrosis is usually more smoothly marginated as opposed to intracystic malignancies and appears to resolve on serial scans.

e) (F) Options b and c are correct.

# References

Doshi DJ, March DE, Crisi GM, Coughlin BF. Complex cystic breast masses: diagnostic approach and imaging-pathologic correlation. Radiographics 2007;27(Suppl 1): S53–S64

Kopans DB. Breast imaging. 3rd ed. Hagerstwon, MD: Lippincott Williams & Wilkins; 2007

*Answer 6:*

| a) | Skin. |
|---|---|
| b) | Mammary layer. |
| c) | Pectoralis muscle. |
| d) | Rib. |

# Reference

Spratt JD, Salkowski LR, Loukas M, et al. Weir & Abrahams' Imaging Atlas of Human Anatomy. 5th ed. Elsevier; 2016

*Answer 7:*

a) (T) Fat necrosis is an entirely benign condition used to describe an injury of the fatty tissue and can occur following trauma, radiation, or surgery.

b) (T) Intracystic malignancy of the breast and fat necrosis can have shared imaging features as both entities can have solid and cystic components. Fat necrosis will not show any flow on Doppler applications.

c) (F) Diabetic mastopathy and lymphocytic mastopathy represent the same spectrum of histopathological features. Lymphocytic mastopathy can be called diabetic mastopathy in diabetic patients.

d) (F) Sarcoidosis rarely occurs within the breast. This most commonly involves lungs, lymphatic system, or cutaneous tissue.

e) (T) Free silicone may trigger formation of siliconomas and become a rare cause of associated foreign body granulomatous mastitis.

# References

Doshi DJ, March DE, Crisi GM, Coughlin BF. Complex cystic breast masses: diagnostic approach and imaging-pathologic correlation. Radiographics 2007;27(Suppl 1): S53–S64

Kopans DB. Breast imaging. 3rd ed. Hagerstwon, MD: Lippincott Williams & Wilkins; 2007

Pluguez-Turull CW, Nanyes JE, Quintero CJ, et al. Idiopathic granulomatous mastitis: manifestations at multimodality imaging and pitfalls. Radiographics 2018;38: 330–356

*Answer 8:*

a) (F) BI-RADS 5 category means highly suspicious for malignancy.

b) (F) BI-RADS 1 category is consistent with a normal result.

c) (T) BI-RADS 2 category means benign findings.

d) (F) BI-RADS 4 category is reserved for lesions that are sufficiently suspicious and require biopsy.

# References

D'Orsi CJ, Sickles EA, Ellen B; American College of Radiology. ACR BI-RADS Atlas der Mammadiagnostik. Berlin, Germany: Springer; 2016

Kopans DB. Breast imaging. 3rd ed. Hagerstwon, MD: Lippincott Williams & Wilkins; 2007

Shah BA, Mandawa SR. Breast Imaging A Core Review. 2nd ed. Philadelphia, PA: Wolters Kluwer; 2017

## Answer 9

a)   (F) No air outlining or halo sign seen.

b)   (F) No radiating structure with spicules is visualized.

c)   (F) Solitary dense mass with mild spicules seen.

d)   (F) No calcifications identified.

e)   (T) The lesion has mild spicules. Structural elements cannot be seen through the mass in keeping with high density mass.

# Reference

Tabar L, Dean PB. Teaching Atlas of Mammography. 4th ed. Thieme; 2011

## Answer 10:

a)   (F) Biopsy is required to exclude malignancy.

b)   (T) An irregular and hypoechoic lesion is visualized. Ultrasound-guided core needle biopsy is the preferred next diagnostic step, as microscopic verification is needed to establish the final diagnosis.

c)   (F) A solid mass on ultrasound is not an indication for MRI.

d)   (F) Stereotactic biopsy could be an option with regard to a mammographic abnormality.

e)   (F) This is a solid mass. No fluid to aspirate identified.

# References

Kopans DB. Breast imaging. 3rd ed. Hagerstwon, MD: Lippincott Williams & Wilkins; 2007

Shah BA, Mandawa SR. Breast Imaging A Core Review. 2nd ed. Philadelphia, PA: Wolters Kluwer; 2017

# Summary Quiz

# Summary Quiz

**Learning Objectives:**

1. To summarize various subgroups of breast cancer mimics and sharpen your skills regarding most appropriate management.

2. To review and describe challenging entities that mislead dedicated breast imagers, list potential imaging features, and discover your strengths in correct recognition.

3. To motivate you to identify potential breast cancer mimics, in relation to clinical history, and gain confidence with regard to interpretation of basic imaging patterns on sonography.

*We hope that new knowledge will empower you and set you up for success in daily practice.*

## Summary MCQs

### ■ Questions

Please choose true or false. More than one answer options may be correct.

*Question 1:* Which of the following statements are correct?

a) Diabetic mastopathy is a common cause of breast cancer.

b) Diabetic mastopathy is not associated with breast malignancy.

c) Long-standing diabetes predisposes to formation of palpable breast masses.

d) Wide local excision is the optimal treatment regarding diabetic mastopathy.

e) Lymphocytic and diabetic mastopathy do not share the same histopathological features.

*Question 2:* A young female was referred to triple breast assessment clinic with bilateral progressive and extensive palpable breast masses. Clinical history revealed long-standing and poorly controlled diabetes type 1. Ultrasound images are shown. What is the most likely diagnosis and impact on patient's management?

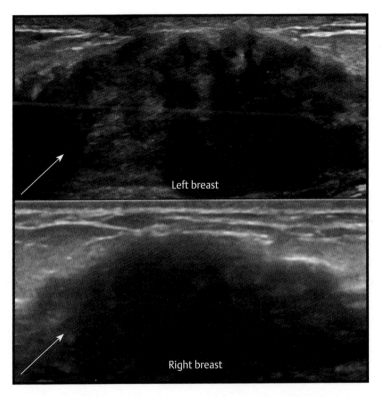

a) Lymphocytic mastopathy in the setting of patient's diabetes and wide local excision as an optimal treatment option.

b) Diabetic mastopathy in the setting of patient's diabetes and wide local excision as an optimal treatment option.

c) Diabetic mastopathy in the setting of patient's diabetes and no surgical treatment required.

d) Lymphocytic mastopathy in the setting of patient's diabetes and no surgical treatment required.

e) Extensive bilateral breast malignancy for baseline magnetic resonance imaging (MRI) to evaluate the total footprint of the disease with a view to neoadjuvant chemotherapy.

**Question 3:** Which of the following statements with regard to giant fibroadenoma are correct?

a) Giant or juvenile fibroadenoma is defined as a fibroadenoma larger than 5 cm.

b) This condition usually presents in elderly patients and causes deformity of the breast.

c) This condition usually presents in adolescents and causes deformity of the breast.

d) Phyllodes tumor is an important differential diagnosis.

e) Giant fibroadenoma is a precancerous condition.

**Question 4:** Ultrasound images of four different patients A to D are shown in the following figure. Which patients are more likely to have breast malignancy and why?

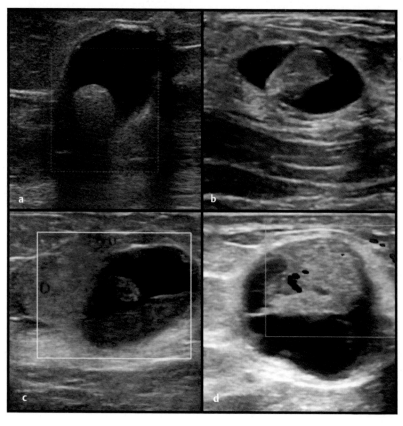

a) Patients A and B are most likely to have a cancer as solid components have no flow on Doppler application.

b) Patients C and D are most likely to have a cancer as there is flow with regard to solid components on Doppler application.

c) All patients have breast cancer as per solid intracystic components.

d) None of the patients has breast malignancy as the images represent benign fibrocystic changes.

e) None of the above is correct.

*Question 5:* A young and healthy patient with a history of trauma was referred to the breast unit with a 1-week history of a new palpable mass. There was no family history of breast malignancy. Ultrasound image is shown. What could be likely differential diagnosis and further management?

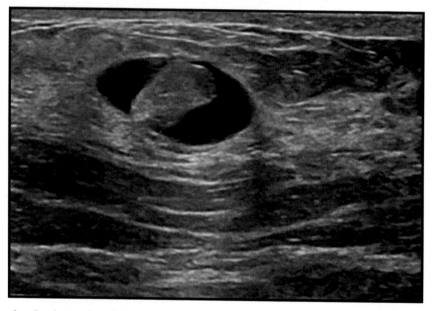

a) Cysticercosis of the breast; patient could benefit from treatment with albendazole.

b) Fibroadenoma; biopsy for confirmation needed.

c) Simple cyst; no further action required.

d) Fat necrosis; follow-up may be considered.

e) Breast cancer; image-guided biopsy required.

**Question 6:** Diabetic mastopathy is shown. Please connect arrows with correct anatomic structures on ultrasound.

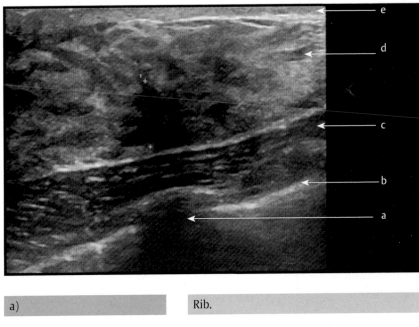

a)          Rib.

b)          Pleura.

c)          Pectoralis muscle.

d)          Fibrofatty breast tissue.

e)          Skin.

*Question 7:* How would you describe the presented mammographic abnormality?

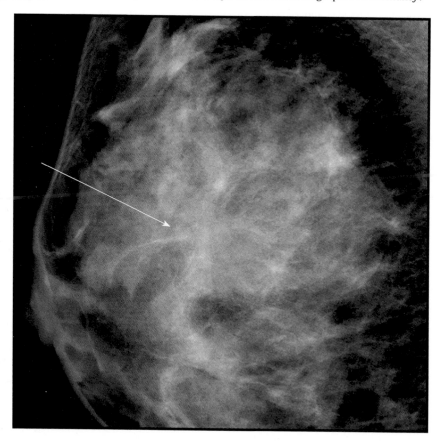

a) Suspicious microcalcifications.

b) Ill-defined, high-density lesion.

c) Lobulated, low-density lesion.

d) Oval, sharply defined lesion

e) Architectural distortion.

*Question 8:* Female patient presented with a palpable breast abnormality. Ultrasound image is shown. What would be the most likely diagnosis based on imaging alone and why?

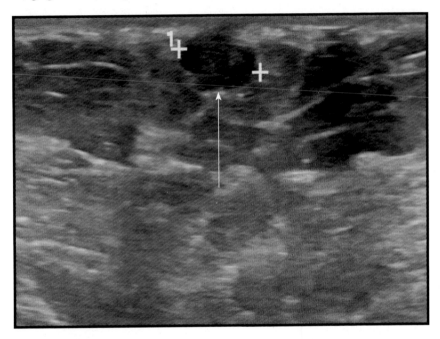

a)  Breast carcinoma.

b)  Fat necrosis.

c)  Sebaceous cyst.

d)  Subcutaneous lipoma.

e)  Simple cyst.

*Question 9:* Cold abscess in the setting of biopsy-proven mammary tuberculosis is shown. Please see ultrasound (*arrow*) and associated histology (*inset*). What would be the best management for the patient?

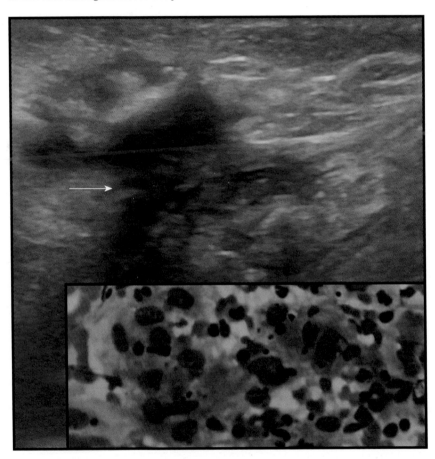

a) Wide local excision with axillary clearance.

b) Treatment regimen with antituberculosis drugs.

c) Radiotherapy.

d) No treatment required as tuberculous mastitis is a self-limiting process.

e) Corticosteroids.

**Question 10:** Sonography and mammography images of a palpable mass are shown. Ultrasound of the axilla was normal. What would be the most appropriate next step?

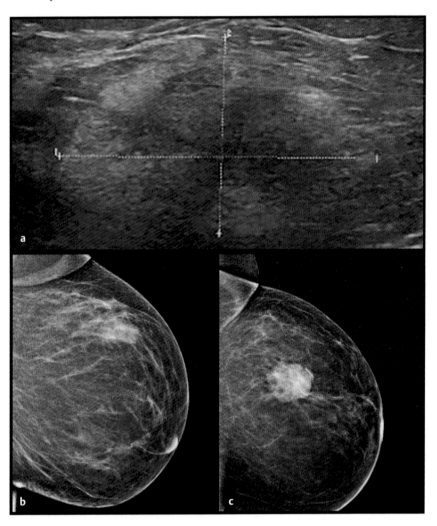

a) Computed tomography (CT) staging.

b) Stereo-guided biopsy.

c) No further action required.

d) MRI.

e) Ultrasound-guided biopsy.

**Question 11:** Based on histology, diagnosis of mammary angiomatosis was made. What would be the final breast imaging reporting and database system (BI-RADS) category?

a)  BI-RADS 5.

b)  BI-RADS 1.

c)  BI-RADS 2.

d)  BI-RADS 4.

e)  BI-RADS 6.

**Question 12:** Which statements with regard to complex cystic lesions of the breast are correct?

a)  Mucinous carcinoma or intracystic papillary carcinoma can present as complex cystic masses.

b)  Doppler application can be helpful in distinguishing benign complex cystic mass from malignancy.

c)  Complex cystic lesions contain both solid-appearing and fluid-like components.

d)  Chronic collections such as postoperative seromas or abscesses can mimic intracystic malignancy.

e)  All of the above.

**Question 13:** Biopsy-proven granular cell tumor of the breast is demonstrated. How would you describe the sonographic findings? And what would be the further management?

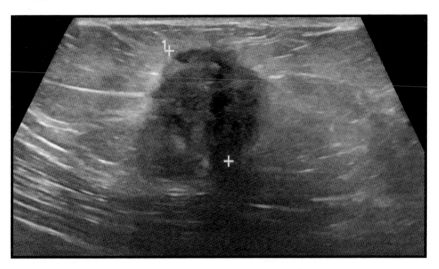

a) Round solid mass.

b) Irregular solid mass.

c) Complex cystic lesion.

d) Smoothly marginated lesion.

e) Oval-shaped lesion with calcifications.

**Question 14:** Which information with regard to hamartoma is correct? Please see ultrasound image below:

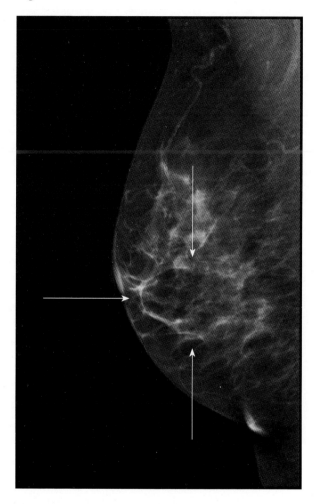

a) Hamartoma is a benign "breast within the breast" lesion that resembles normal breast.

b) Fibroadenolipoma is a synonymous medical descriptor.

c) This condition has malignant potential and increases risk of breast cancer.

d) Mammography usually shows both radiolucent fatty components and dense glandular tissue.

e) There is strong association with breast cancer.

**Question 15:** Example of a radial scar is illustrated. How would you describe the presented mammographic findings?

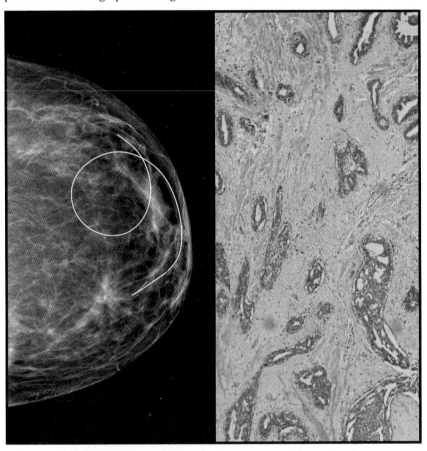

a) Oval lesion with mixed density.

b) Stellate/spiculated lesion.

c) No significant mammographic abnormality identified.

d) Oval radiolucent lesion.

e) Lobulated, high-density lesion.

*Question 16:* Which information with regard to radial scar/complex sclerosing lesion is correct? More options are possible.

a)   Radial scar is a benign proliferative lesion which mimics breast carcinoma.

b)   This resembles postoperative fat necrosis and contains coarse calcifications on mammography.

c)   Radial scar usually presents as a spiculate stellate lesion on mammography.

d)   Fibroadenoma and a radial scar have similar imaging features.

e)   Radial scar is a high-risk breast lesion.

*Question 17:* Sonography and histology images of pseudoangiomatous stromal hyperplasia (PASH) are demonstrated. Which information with regard to this entity is correct? More options are possible.

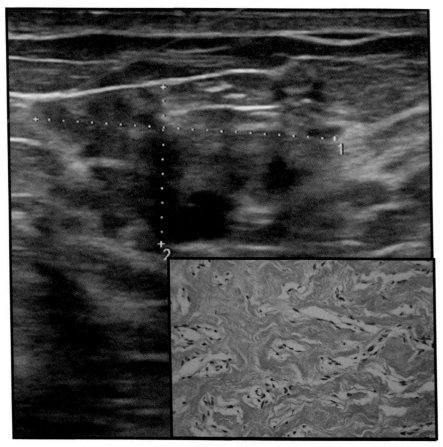

a)  PASH is a noncancerous lesion.

b)  PASH is a precancerous lesion.

c)  PASH is a high-risk lesion.

d)  This condition requires wide local excision.

e)  This condition is benign and does not require any treatment.

**Question 18:** What potential conditions or diseases could predispose to the development of breast granulomas?

a)  Sarcoidosis.

b)  Silicone injections.

c)  Granulomatosis with polyangiitis, formerly known as Wegener's granulomatosis.

d)  Diabetic mastopathy.

e)  Hashimoto thyroiditis.

**Question 19:** Parasitic infestation of the breast in the setting of filariasis is demonstrated. Please see ultrasound and histology images below. Which ultrasound features and clinical information could guide us to such diagnosis?

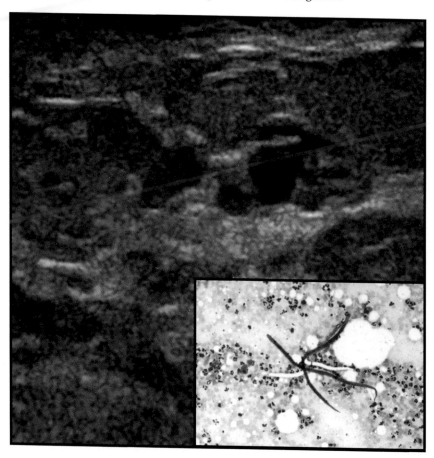

a) Slow-growing, painful mass in a female from the subtropical region.

b) Painful mass in a diabetic patient with high body mass index (BMI).

c) Complex cystic lesion with rapid-moving contents in endemic area.

d) New palpable mass in a patient with Hashimoto thyroiditis.

e) Chronic abscess in a female with a history of pulmonary tuberculosis.

*Question 20:* What potential clinical scenario could guide us to the diagnosis of breast cancer mimics?

a)   A 30-year old female with a history of long-standing diabetes type 1 presents with a palpably hard mass.

b)   A 45-year old woman with a history of relapse of sarcoidosis presents with multiple palpable nodules within the breast.

c)   Immunosuppressed patient with history of tuberculosis presents with a new complex cystic lesion within the breast.

d)   BRCA-positive patient who is referred to the breast unit with a new breast lump.

e)   A young female with a seatbelt injury presents with a new large lump within the breast.

# ■ Answers

*Answer 1:*

a)   (F) Diabetic mastopathy is not associated with breast cancer.

b)   (T) Diabetic mastopathy is not associated with breast malignancy. This is an entirely benign condition which does not increase the risk of developing breast cancer.

c)   (T) Long-standing diabetes predisposes to formation of palpable breast masses. Chronic diabetes results in fibrosis of fibrofatty tissue and subsequent palpable mass formation.

d)   (F) Diabetic mastopathy is entirely benign and does not require surgery.

e)   (F) Lymphocytic and diabetic mastopathy share the same spectrum of histopathological features.

# References

Kopans DB. Breast imaging. 3rd ed. Hagerstwon, MD: Lippincott Williams & Wilkins; 2007

Pluguez-Turull CW, Nanyes JE, Quintero CJ, et al. Idiopathic granulomatous mastitis: manifestations at multimodality imaging and pitfalls. Radiographics 2018;38(2): 330–356

Shah BA, Mandawa SR. Breast Imaging A Core Review. 2nd ed. Philadelphia, PA: Wolters Kluwer; 2017

*Answer 2:*

a)  (F) Lymphocytic mastopathy in the setting of patient's diabetes is the diagnosis. However, this is a benign condition and no surgical treatment is required. Medical descriptors, lymphocytic or diabetic mastopathy, can be used synonymously in diabetic patients.

b)  (F) Diabetic mastopathy in the setting of patient's diabetes is the appropriate diagnosis. However, this is a benign condition and no surgical treatment is required. Medical descriptors, lymphocytic or diabetic mastopathy, can be used synonymously regarding diabetic patients.

c)  (T) Diabetic mastopathy in the setting of patient's diabetes and no surgical treatment is required. Medical descriptors, lymphocytic or diabetic mastopathy, can be used synonymously in diabetic patients.

d)  (T) Lymphocytic mastopathy in the setting of patient's diabetes and no surgical treatment is required. Medical descriptors, lymphocytic or diabetic mastopathy, can be used synonymously in diabetic patients.

e)  (F) These are benign breast cancer mimics in the setting of long-standing diabetes and no invasive treatment is required.

## References

Kopans DB. Breast imaging. 3rd ed. Hagerstwon, MD: Lippincott Williams & Wilkins; 2007

Pluguez-Turull CW, Nanyes JE, Quintero CJ, et al. Idiopathic granulomatous mastitis: manifestations at multimodality imaging and pitfalls. Radiographics 2018;38(2): 330–356

Shah BA, Mandawa SR. Breast Imaging A Core Review. 2nd ed. Philadelphia, PA: Wolters Kluwer; 2017

*Answer 3:*

a)  (T) Giant or juvenile fibroadenoma is defined as a fibroadenoma larger than 5 cm.

b)  (F) This condition usually presents in adolescents and may cause deformity of the breast.

c)  (T) This condition usually presents in adolescents and causes deformity of the breast.

d)  (T) Phyllodes tumor is an important differential diagnosis.

e)   (F) Giant fibroadenoma is a benign condition and does not increase risk of malignancy.

## References

Ikeda DM, Miyake KK. Breast Imaging: The Requisites. 3rd ed. St Louis, MO: Elsevier; 2017

Kopans DB. Breast imaging. 3rd ed. Hagerstwon, MD: Lippincott Williams & Wilkins; 2007

*Answer 4:*

a)   (F) Patients A and B are less likely to have a cancer than patients C and D, as solid components have no flow on Doppler application.

b)   (T) Patients C and D are most likely to have a cancer as there is flow with regard to solid components on Doppler application.

c)   (F) Not necessarily, as benign mimics such as fat necrosis or inflammatory conditions can present as complex lesions with both solid-appearing and fluid-like components.

d)   (F) Patients C and D are highly suspicious for intracystic malignancy as there is flow with regard to solid components on Doppler application.

e)   (F) Patients C and D are most likely to have a cancer, as there is flow with regard to solid components on Doppler application. Option b is correct.

## References

Ikeda DM, Miyake KK. Breast Imaging: The Requisites. 3rd ed. St Louis, MO: Elsevier; 2017

Kopans DB. Breast imaging. 3rd ed. Hagerstwon, MD: Lippincott Williams & Wilkins; 2007

*Answer 5:*

a)   (F) Clinical history is suggestive of posttraumatic change, and ultrasound illustrates smoothly marginated complex lesion typical for fat necrosis. There is no correlating history that would suggest parasitic infestation of the breast.

b)   (F) Typical fibroadenoma is entirely solid and does not contain fluid-like components.

c)   (F) This is not a simple cyst as contains solid-appearing components.

d) (T) Fat necrosis represents benign posttraumatic change. Fat necrosis represents benign posttraumatic change which may resolve on serial scans. Follow-up may be considered.

e) (F) Breast cancer appears less likely in the view of the clinical history.

## References

Kopans DB. Breast imaging. 3rd ed. Hagerstwon, MD: Lippincott Williams & Wilkins; 2007

Ikeda DM, Miyake KK. Breast Imaging: The Requisites. 3rd ed. St Louis, MO: Elsevier; 2017

Tabar L, Dean PB. Teaching Atlas of Mammography. 4th ed. Thieme; 2011

*Answer 6:*

| a) | Rib. |
|---|---|
| b) | Pleura. |
| c) | Pectoralis muscle. |
| d) | Fibrofatty breast tissue. |
| e) | Skin. |

## Reference

Spratt JD, Salkowski LR, Loukas M, et al. Weir & Abrahams' Imaging Atlas of Human Anatomy. 5th ed. Elsevier; 2016

*Answer 7:*

a) (No) There are no microcalcifications. Stellate lesion/distortion seen.

b) (No) No overt, high-density mass identified. Subtle stellate lesion in keeping with distortion visualized.

c) (No) No lobulated lesion seen. Subtle, stellate lesion in keeping with distortion visualized.

d) (No) No sharply defined lesion identified. Subtle stellate lesion in keeping with distortion visualized.

e) (Yes) Subtle stellate/spiculate lesion in keeping with architectural distortion noted.

## Reference

Tabar L, Dean PB. Teaching Atlas of Mammography. 4th ed. Thieme; 2011

### Answer 8

a) (No) No evidence of breast carcinoma. Ultrasound shows typical superficial sebaceous cyst with a small sinus tract formation. See *black arrow* in the image below.

b) (No) Fat necrosis usually presents as cystic or complex cystic lesions. This is a purely solid lesion.

c) (Yes) Ultrasound illustrates typical features of subcutaneous sebaceous cyst (*white arrow*), with characteristic sinus tract extending toward the skin (*black arrow*).

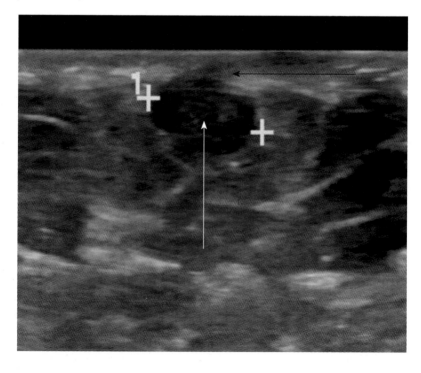

d) (No) Subcutaneous lipoma would have more benign appearance and most frequently present as hyperechoic or isoechoic ovoid lesion.

e) (No) No simple cyst identified. Typical sonographic features of a sebaceous cyst noted.

## Reference

Ikeda DM, Miyake KK. Breast Imaging: The Requisites. 3rd ed. St Louis, MO: Elsevier; 2017

*Answer 9:*

a) (No) Wide local excision with axillary clearance is not required. Antituberculous treatment is the first line of treatment.

b) (Yes) Treatment regimen with antituberculosis drugs required.

c) (No) Radiotherapy is not required. Antituberculous treatment is the first line of treatment.

d) (No) Antituberculous treatment is required as tuberculous mastitis, unlike idiopathic granulomatous mastitis, is not a self-limiting process.

e) (No) Corticosteroids may worsen the symptoms. Antituberculous treatment is the first line of treatment.

## References

Kopans DB. Breast imaging. 3rd ed. Hagerstwon, MD: Lippincott Williams & Wilkins; 2007

Pluguez-Turull CW, Nanyes JE, Quintero CJ, et al. Idiopathic granulomatous mastitis: manifestations at multimodality imaging and pitfalls. Radiographics 2018;38(2): 330–356

*Answer 10:*

a) (No) CT staging is reserved for patients with biopsy-proven cancer.

b) (No) Stereo-guided biopsy is not optimal solution, as the main target is easily visualised with ultrasound. In addition, ultrasound-guided biopsy is the preferred option due to lack of radiation.

c) (No) Ultrasound-guided biopsy is required in order to exclude malignant process.

d) (No) Solitary mass on mammogram, and ultrasound is not an indication for MRI.

e) (Yes) Ultrasound-guided biopsy is the preferred next diagnostic step as malignancy needs to be excluded.

## Reference

Shah BA, Mandawa SR. Breast Imaging A Core Review. 2nd ed. Philadelphia, PA: Wolters Kluwer; 2017

*Answer 11*

a) (F) BI-RADS 5 category means highly suspicious for malignancy.

b) (F) BI-RADS 1 category is consistent with a normal result.

c) (T) BI-RADS 2 category means benign findings.

d) (F) BI-RADS 4 category is reserved for lesions that are not typical of malignancy but are sufficiently suspicious and require biopsy.

e) (F) BI-RADS 6 category is reserved for biopsy-proven breast malignancy.

## References

D'Orsi CJ, Sickles EA, Ellen B; American College of Radiology. ACR BI-RADS Atlas der Mammadiagnostik. Berlin, Germany: Springer; 2016

Kopans DB. Breast imaging. 3rd ed. Hagerstwon, MD: Lippincott Williams & Wilkins; 2007

Shah BA, Mandawa SR. Breast Imaging A Core Review. 2nd ed. Philadelphia, PA: Wolters Kluwer; 2017

*Answer 12:*

a) (T) Mucinous carcinoma or intracystic papillary carcinoma can present as complex cystic masses.

b) (T) Doppler application can be helpful in distinguishing benign complex cystic mass from malignancy. This can demonstrate flow within solid-appearing components in case of carcinoma.

c) (T) Complex cystic lesions contain both solid-appearing and fluid-like components.

d) (T) Chronic collections such as postoperative seromas or abscesses can mimic intracystic malignancy.

e) (T) All options are correct.

# References

Ikeda DM, Miyake KK. Breast Imaging: The Requisites. 3rd ed. St Louis, MO: Elsevier; 2017

Kopans DB. Breast imaging. 3rd ed. Hagerstwon, MD: Lippincott Williams & Wilkins; 2007

Shah BA, Mandawa SR. Breast Imaging A Core Review. 2nd ed. Philadelphia, PA: Wolters Kluwer; 2017

**Answer 13:**

a)  (F) This solid mass is irregular in shape.

b)  (T) Irregular, solid mass noted.

c)  (F) This is an irregular, solid mass and does not have any cystic component.

d)  (F) This is not a smoothly marginated lesion and has irregular shape.

e)  (F) This is not an oval-shaped lesion and no calcifications are identified. The presented mass is irregular in shape.

# References

Kopans DB. Breast imaging. 3rd ed. Hagerstwon, MD: Lippincott Williams & Wilkins; 2007

Tabar L, Dean PB. Teaching Atlas of Mammography. 4th ed. Thieme; 2011

**Answer 14:**

a)  (T) Hamartoma is a benign "breast within the breast" lesion that resembles normal breast.

b)  (T) Fibroadenolipoma is a synonymous medical descriptor.

c)  (F) This condition has no malignant potential and does not increase the risk of breast cancer.

d)  (T) Mammography usually shows both radiolucent fatty components and dense glandular tissue.

e)  (F) There no association with breast malignancy.

# References

Ikeda DM, Miyake KK. Breast Imaging: The Requisites. 3rd ed. St Louis, MO: Elsevier; 2017

Kopans DB. Breast imaging. 3rd ed. Hagerstwon, MD: Lippincott Williams & Wilkins; 2007

*Answer 15:*

a)  (F) No oval lesion identified. Stellate/spiculated lesion noted.

b)  (T) Stellate/spiculated lesion seen.

c)  (F) Stellate/spiculated lesion noted.

d)  (F) No oval radiolucent lesion seen. Stellate/spiculated lesion noted.

e)  (F) No lobulated, high-density lesion seen. Stellate/spiculated lesion noted.

## Reference

Tabar L, Dean PB. Teaching Atlas of Mammography. 4th ed. Thieme; 2011

*Answer 16:*

a)  (T) Radial scar is a benign proliferative lesion which mimics breast carcinoma.

b)  (F) This usually presents as a stellate lesion and does not contain coarse calcifications on mammography.

c)  (T) Radial scar usually presents as a spiculate, stellate lesion on mammography.

d)  (F) Fibroadenoma and a radial scar do not possess any similar imaging features, as radial scar usually presents as a spiculate, stellate lesion on mammography. Fibroadenoma usually presents as a well-defined mass on both mammography and ultrasound.

e)  (T) Radial scar is a high-risk breast lesion.

## References

Ikeda DM, Miyake KK. Breast Imaging: The Requisites. 3rd ed. St Louis, MO: Elsevier; 2017

Kopans DB. Breast imaging. 3rd ed. Hagerstwon, MD: Lippincott Williams & Wilkins; 2007

*Answer 17:*

a)  (T) PASH is a purely benign entity.

b)  (F) PASH is not a precancerous lesion.

c)  (F) PASH is not a high-risk lesion and does not increase the risk of developing breast cancer.

d)  (F) This condition is entirely benign and does not require wide local excision.

e)  (T) This condition is benign and does not require any treatment.

# Reference

Kopans DB. Breast imaging. 3rd ed. Hagerstwon, MD: Lippincott Williams & Wilkins; 2007

*Answer 18:*

a) (T) Mammary sarcoidosis can manifest as breast nodules in the setting of sarcoid granulomas.

b) (T) Silicone injections predispose to foreign body granulomas formation.

c) (T) Granulomatosis with polyangiitis (formerly known as Wegener's granulomatosis) may lead to granulomas formation. Manifestation in the breast is rare.

d) (F) Diabetic mastopathy is not related to granulomatous diseases of the breast.

e) (F) Hashimoto thyroiditis not related to granulomatous diseases of the breast. This condition may be associated with lymphocytic mastopathy.

# References

Kopans DB. Breast imaging. 3rd ed. Hagerstwon, MD: Lippincott Williams & Wilkins; 2007

Pluguez-Turull CW, Nanyes JE, Quintero CJ, et al. Idiopathic granulomatous mastitis: manifestations at multimodality imaging and pitfalls. Radiographics 2018;38(2): 330–356

*Answer 19:*

a) (T) Slow-growing, painful mass in a female from subtropical region raises possibility of parasitic infestation as a differential diagnosis.

b) (F) Painful mass in a diabetic patient with high BMI is suggestive of an abscess as diabetes predisposes to infective mastitis.

c) (T) Complex cystic lesion with rapid moving contents in endemic area would be highly suspicious for "filarial dance" in the setting of mammary filariasis.

d) (F) New palpable mass in a patient with Hashimoto thyroiditis raises suspicion of lymphocytic mastopathy with subsequent palpable mass formation.

e) (F) Chronic abscess in a female with a history of pulmonary tuberculosis is concerning for cold abscess in the setting of tuberculous mastitis.

## References

Chapparia P, Singh C, Mathur N, Sharoff L. Case 12724 Filariasis in breast - Realtime US for solving this clinical dilemma. Eurorad Radiological Case Database; https://www. eurorad.org/case/12724

Pluguez-Turull CW, Nanyes JE, Quintero CJ, et al. Idiopathic granulomatous mastitis: manifestations at multimodality imaging and pitfalls. Radiographics 2018;38(2): 330–356

*Answer 20:*

a) (T) A 30-year old female with a history of long-standing diabetes type 1 presents with a palpably hard mass. This is highly suggestive of palpable mass in the setting of patient's diabetic mastopathy.

b) (T) A 45-year old woman with a history of relapse of sarcoidosis presents with multiple palpable nodules within the breast. Clinical history is highly suggestive of mammary sarcoidosis and associated granulomas.

c) (T) Immunosuppressed patient with history of tuberculosis presents with a new complex cystic lesion within the breast. This clinical scenario raises suspicion of mammary tuberculosis and cold abscess formation.

d) (F) History of BRCA-positive patient who is referred to the breast unit with a new breast lump is concerning for a breast carcinoma.

e) (T) A young female with a seatbelt injury presents with a new large lump within the breast. This scenario is typical for subsequent posttraumatic changes and fat necrosis.

## References

Kopans DB. Breast imaging. 3rd ed. Hagerstwon, MD: Lippincott Williams & Wilkins; 2007

Pluguez-Turull CW, Nanyes JE, Quintero CJ, et al. Idiopathic granulomatous mastitis: manifestations at multimodality imaging and pitfalls. Radiographics 2018;38(2): 330–356

# Index